T0162829

Beyond Weight Loss

*The Complete Weight
Management Program*

Althea A. Madden, CNP

iUniverse LLC
Bloomington

BEYOND WEIGHT LOSS
THE COMPLETE WEIGHT MANAGEMENT PROGRAM

iUniverse books may be ordered through booksellers or by contacting:

iUniverse
1663 Liberty Drive
Bloomington, IN 47403
www.iuniverse.com
1-800-Authors (1-800-288-4677)

ISBN: 978-1-4917-1559-8 (sc)
ISBN: 978-1-4917-1560-4 (hc)
ISBN: 978-1-4917-1561-1 (e)

Library of Congress Control Number: 2013920849

Printed in the United States of America.

iUniverse rev. date: 1/14/2014

Beyond Weight Loss is dedicated to Enid, Roselda, and Landy Madden, who have taught me the value of perseverance. Without the three of you, this book would not have been possible.

CONTENTS

Introduction... ix

1 Weight and Health...1
   The Weight of It All   1
   Self First   5
   Guilt and Obligation   11
   Emotional Connection   21
   Stress Meter   33
   The Weight of Moving   38
   Fitness   49

2 Weight and Career..55
   Searching for Purpose   55
   Life Lessons   57
   Life Passion   70
   Elements of Career Satisfaction   83

3 Weight and Money 99
   The Money-Weight Connection   99
   The Money-Weight Message   119

4 Weight and Relationships 127
   Self   128
   Romance   130
   Friendships   133
   Acquaintances   140
   Working Relationships   144
   Family Dynamics   147
   Food   151

5 Weight and Home 154
   Belonging   154
   Home Sweet Home   159
   Organized Space   168

6 Weight and Growth 170
   Personal Growth and Development   170
   Conflict for Growth   175
   Energy Zappers   187
   Teachers in Disguise   190

7 Weight and Spirituality 199
   What Is Spirituality?   199
   Internal Guidance System   200
   Look Within   207
   The Best Teacher   213

Conclusion 219

INTRODUCTION

Just before the release of my first book, *Weight Loss for Life*, I was telling someone about it and how I felt like a fraud. I was avoiding promoting the book because I was gaining the weight back. Why was this happening to me at this moment? Maya Angelou said, "You do better when you know better." I believed at the time I knew better, so why was I regaining this weight that had taken me so long to lose? I felt that all my hard work was a waste of time. Now what was I to do? I continued to explore why I was still in the same position despite being an "expert" in this area.

I believed that this happened because that was not the book for me to write. Don't get me wrong—it's an amazing book that I love, and I am very proud of it. What I'm saying is the focus must be off losing weight and onto the *management* of one's weight on a daily basis. Just like me, you do know how to lose weight. People do it day in and day out on diets that are sometimes healthy and sometimes unhealthy. You are also an expert. What we lack are the tools for keeping it off.

This book is about discovering what makes you happy, content, and fulfiled; compiling an action plan; and executing that plan. This process is how you will manage your weight. By following the program, your obsessive behaviours about food and your body will be channelled into something more positive. It's about doing what you love, feel passionate about, and have fun doing.

Now, let's start off by being absolutely real about everything that's going on within and around you and is contributing to this condition. Ask yourself, *How many diets have I been on in the past week, month, year, and five years? How much weight have I lost in this period, only to gain it back?* I have been on a diet almost every day since I was 13 years old. I have tried most of the popular diets on the market today; some worked and some didn't. Then, just like millions of other women, I would gain the weight back. What this has done for me is make me an expert in weight loss.

Weight loss has not changed over the years: it's about eating nutrient-rich foods based on your physical and mental needs and desires and then participating in physical activities that you enjoy. Yes, you know how to lose weight because you've done it over and over, year after year. What's missing is the knowledge of how to manage this process in a healthy, sustainable way for the rest of your life.

Based on my personal experience and work as a coach and nutritional consultant, I've come to understand that managing our weight is 25 percent diet, 25 percent exercise, and 50 percent balancing your life. I call the management portion "The Seven Success Factors to Weight Management." Losing weight and keeping it off involves bringing balance to the seven key areas of your life. I know what you're thinking—it's easier said than done. I'm here to tell you that it's not. All you have to do is take the first step, and the rest will fall into place with ease. You may think, *So, Althea, are you saying I'm fat because I'm out of balance in one or more of these areas?* Yes, absolutely.

As mentioned earlier, most of us who have been on a diet

do know what to eat to remain strong, lean, and healthy. So why are we not doing so? It has nothing to do with physical health and everything to do with the avoidance of pain. The question then becomes how we can avoid pain and live a strong, lean, and healthy lifestyle. We only have to do one thing, and that's bring balance to our lives in seven key areas, which I call life centres: career, financial support, health and fitness, relationships, home, personal growth and development, and spirituality.

The Healthea Solutions Weight Management Program consists of five simple steps to balancing your seven life centres. It's my belief that living a balanced life results in a balanced diet and permanent weight management. In this book you will learn to do the following:

1. **Identify imbalance:** Which life centres are out of balance?
2. **Identify causes of imbalance:** What core beliefs, attitudes, and behaviours are associated with the storage of excess body fat in each life centre?
3. **Bring yourself into balance:** personal wants, needs, and desires.
4. **Establish an action plan** for achieving success.
5. **Follow up and maintain** the plan of action.

After reading this book, please drop me a line at aam@ healtheasolutions.ca. I'm anxious to hear what you think of this book and how you will use it to manage your life.

Happy reading!
Much love,
Althea

WEIGHT AND HEALTH

The Weight of It All

The road map for self-healing is within you. As a weight management coach, my job is simple: to guide you in accessing your natural ability to heal from the inside out. I show you how to be happy and healthy with and within yourself. Erase the old self-sabotage programs placed in your mind by individuals in your childhood. Who placed those bad programs there? They are seeds that were planted in your head and are keeping you from being healthy, happy, and successful today. By recognizing what and where they are, you can begin to accept them and start the healing process.

There are seven chapters in this book, and this one is by far the most important to my personal survival. This is the one subject that has been eluding me for the past several years. I do know that I turn to food to avoid pain. At the start of writing this chapter, I still did not understand why I chose food. There are so many other ways to avoid feeling hurt, so why was I insisting on sticking to that which I knew did not have my best interests at heart? Why did I continue to eat foods that were dangerous to my health?

What is health? What contributes to poor health? What are the key components for optimal health? What are the effects of weight on health? What's the best health plan for me? In this chapter we will explore these and many other questions, ensuring we all have a clear understanding of how being overweight affects our overall health. I believe that in order to make a healthy permanent change, we must first understand our behaviours.

As mentioned in my first book, *Weight Loss for Life,* I have been concerned about my weight since the age of 13. As a result I have tried most fad diets on the market today, and yes, they all worked for me. The problem is that I was not able to maintain the permanent weight loss we all want—until now. Today, managing my weight is not an issue because I no longer go on diets. I finally realized that staying on that weight-loss roller coaster would lead me to an early grave. This is the opposite of why I first got into the health field: to save my own life.

It all started on September 2, 1997, when my healthy mom went to bed and did not wake up. She was only 51 years old and was in reasonably good health. After the funeral I was obsessed with living a long and healthy life. I then left my well-paying job to go back to school and study nutrition. After completing the program, I realized that part of the puzzle was still missing. After much research I realized that the reason I was still struggling with my weight was because of my hidden, unexpressed emotions. These are the thoughts and feelings that I have been hiding from for years, though they were hidden in plain sight. I disguised them as something else. For example, after 3:00 p.m. I would turn to processed food instead of taking a nap because my body craved rest. At work when I was angry, I would ingest high-calorie coffee drinks instead of acknowledging my feelings of being stuck. I was in retail, a profession that I knew was not right for me, and I was having difficulty transitioning into the health field, which was where I desperately wanted to be. Health was a field where I could help women on a deeper level, guiding them to live happy, strong, lean, healthy, and balanced lives.

Over the years I've learned that my food cravings were always telling me what my body needed in order to live a long, lean, and healthy life free of pain, aches, and diseases. We are overweight because we use food as medication to cover up and suppress our past hurts and feelings, as well as what direction we should take. As humans we are hard-wired to avoid pain and seek pleasure. This chapter focuses on health and not weight loss, because I believe when we experience optimal health, our weight will not be an issue.

Many times I've been asked what the secret to weight loss is, and I say it's very simple: there is no secret to losing weight. Things have not changed over the years; it's the same today as it was centuries ago in that all we have to do is burn off more calories than we take in. There are no new ways, only recycled concepts with a new spin. The only thing that has changed for this millennium is making sure we eat less packaged foods and more natural ones if possible.

What *has* changed is how to keep the weight off. Instead of focusing on weight loss, we must instead focus on what we should do to maintain our weight on a daily basis. We must look at and determine which life centre is out of balance. We should determine personal wants, needs, and desire and then act on them. It's about identifying the root causes of our unhappiness. If we focus on what we need to be healthy in mind, body, and spirit, the weight will normalize itself.

Congratulations—you've lost the weight! You are finally at your goal weight, and you look and feel amazing. Now, how are you going to *keep* the weight off? Writing away my weight, along with studying and teaching weight management, is what works for me. This is how I will continue maintaining my strong, lean, and healthy body for the rest of my life. The other part of my plan is to travel to spiritual retreats and spas throughout the world, learning and experiencing the different healing modalities. I'm starting here in Vancouver and am working my way outword and upword. To be happy you must have a goal, something to work toward.

How did I come to this conclusion? Keep reading and find out. To start, I've lost and regained much too much weight over the years. Three times I lost more than 65 pounds each time. After years of searching for my reason for this weight gain, I've come up with this hypothesis: Living on purpose inspires us. When we are feeling inspired, we eat nutrient-rich food that nourishes our mind, body, and spirit. It's about living the life we are here to live. So what does this mean?

Let's look at what you are passionate about. What is the one thing you want more than anything else in the world? What is the one thing at which others have been saying you would excel! This has to be something that you are good at, that you enjoy doing, and that comes naturally to you. It may also be the one thing in this world that scares you the most.

There are likely lots of things you are good at, but you lack passion for the work. You are more likely to stick to it if you are extremely passionate while thinking about it, talking about it, and doing it. You lose track of time doing it, and it replenishes your depleted energy. When you are living on purpose in your life centres, then every decision you make is for your own good. Whatever you do, you must have love for it! If you are doing it out of guilt, obligation, or simply to pay the bills, then it won't work, and you will never be happy living that way. Most important, instead of maintaining a strong, lean, healthy body, you will instead gain more weight, leading to obesity and other life-threatening illnesses that could lead to death.

I believe that we experience specific challenges throughout our lives so that we can get to know our authentic selves— who we are, what we are, and what we do. We learn what's negotiable in our lives and what's not. It's like a baby starting out touching everything, and by the time she gets to be a certain age, she realizes what she likes and what hurts. It's the pleasure-versus-pain scenario.

My focus is on getting beyond weight loss. Once we lose the weight, how do we keep it off? We retain excess body fat because we are out of balance. Maintaining a strong, lean, healthy body involves continually asking ourselves the following three questions: "Where do I see myself? What do I see myself doing? With whom do I see myself doing it?" These questions work in all seven life centres and are even more relevant when it comes to our overall health.

Self First

One of the most important parts of any health plan is taking time out for yourself each and every day, even if it is only five minutes. It's doing what's best for you at all times without question. You must put yourself first on your daily agenda. When you don't, then you tend to get angry and frustrated, and then you turn to food for comfort.

Living life on your own terms is about putting yourself where you want to be, doing what you love, and spending time around people you enjoy. Putting the needs of others ahead of your own can result in feeling lost, isolated, and even resentful toward the people closest to you. Taking the time you need to nurture yourself will lead you to peace, happiness, stabilized weight, and optimal health.

Our excessive body weight is communicating this fact to us. But are we listening to what it's telling us? We are experiencing pain in our lives because we are resisting that which we are, that which we must do! We are the cause of our own pain. Pain is the result of attempting to protect ourselves when we don't need protection. We get hurt whether or not we try to protect ourselves. As a matter of fact, when we don't interfere with the learning process, we experience less pain and get to the learning much quicker.

To know the truth is to be open to happiness. The question then becomes, "What am I protecting myself from? Is it from love because my past has shown me that love hurts?" I am protecting my heart from being broken, which has never worked—in fact, all protection has done is caused me more pain. I therefore surrender to the need to protect myself and instead become wide open to love in all its forms and glory. When you take time out for you, then you can see and understand what's happening to you much clearer.

All challenges, be they mental, emotional, or physical, are opportunities to heal old wounds. Sometimes we get to the point where we believe we have finally understood a particular painful situation, only to have it raise its ugly head again. Why is that? Sometimes we have to go deeper to ensure the wound is completely clean; other times it's a test to see if we have truly let go of this pain attached to a specific event. Have we really learned the lesson, or are we simply saying so?

Your physical body frame always knows where you don't want to be, what you don't want to do, and who you don't want to be around. When you are not listening, then it brings about pain, forcing you to *focus* on a specific action. Here is one such example. On a Sunday and Monday, I finally pushed my body too far, and it reacted by shutting down. I'd worked 13 hours each day. On the Monday I was feeling extremely drained, so at 5:30 p.m. I went for an hour break. After the break I stood up and noticed I was limping. As I walked, I started to feel better. On my way home, I got off the bus and started to limp again, and the sharp pain in the back of my right leg intensified. As I walked, I started to feel better again.

That night I had trouble getting into bed, and I was unable to lie on my right side. It took me forever to turn over. I was uncomfortable on my left side, back, and front as well. The pain was excruciating, throbbing no matter what position I tried. Each time I fell asleep, I would wake up minutes later in tremendous pain.

I waited until the walk-in clinic opened six blocks away and hobbled there. With each step I regretted my decision to walk instead of taking a taxi. When I finally got there, the receptionist told me only two people were in front of me, so I should take a seat. I told her I could not sit down and hobbled over to the corner, where I could support my back by leaning on the wall and standing on my left foot. After about 20 minutes I got in to see the doctor. She asked me a few questions and examined my right upper thigh, and then she told me it was a muscle strain that was affecting the tendons.

I was given the names of two pain medications, a form for having X-rays within a week, and a doctor's note for time off work. I took a cab home, poured a bowl of cereal, sat on the coach, and took the pain medication with breakfast. I was in the same position all day, sleeping while sitting up.

What does all this have to do with weight management? Everything! I worked 26 hours in two days on almost no sleep, and I drank a lot of coffee and did not work out. I was stressing my body with a lack of proper nutrition, exercise, sleep, and rest. Instead, I was feeding it pills to suppress the pain I was in so that I could continue to burn the candle at both ends. I was putting my body into starvation mode.

All this forced me to look at my work ethic. As mentioned earlier, I learned an unrealistic work ethic from two amazingly strong women, my mom and grandmother. These chains of events reminded me that both these women worked their way to an early grave—and if I was not careful, I would do the same. As a result I made the decision to pay close attention to how much time I spent on the job. I also decided that working as hard as I was for only money was counterproductive. It was taking time away from my true passion of studying, writing, and teaching weight management. In that instant I made the decision that I would only work an extra two hours on store merchandising days, which was approximately every three weeks. I would then donate more time to writing. I am sticking to writing for a minimum of 15 minutes daily, and at least once per week for 5 hours straight; that time can include research.

With that said, I wondered what old wounds were attached to my unhealthy eating habits, resulting in weight gain. I paid close attention to what I was doing and to how I was using my energy. I had to take the time to focus on my passion. What I'd been doing did not feed my soul—in fact, it was really draining my energy. It was telling me to listen to the voice within!

Food is nourishment that provides fuel, energy, and stamina. When my mind is being flooded with thoughts of food, it means I'm in need of nourishment. *What part of me needs to be nourished, fueled, energized, and strengthened? What kind of nourishment is needed?* My overweight body is screaming at me, "I'm in pain. Can't you see I need help? Why can't you help me? Why can't you help me save my life today?" Take care of yourself first; make yourself a priority in your own life. You need to be your own parent in this moment and nurture yourself.

Look at how the people in your life are affecting your health. Each person entering into your life does so for a reason: to introduce parts of yourself to you. They are a mirror of your thoughts, actions, and behaviours. When someone is irritating you, mentally ask him or her, "What message or lesson do you have for me today?" or, "How am I acting like you at this moment?" I believe that they are pushing your buttons so that you can get better acquainted with yourself, prompting you to take better care of yourself. They force you to face thoughts, feelings, and behaviours that you are exhibiting as a result of what you are avoiding. Face the music, and the cravings will go away. What comes to the surface is what's been waiting to come out. When it surfaces, you then have a choice to examine the issue or ignore it. In my case, I'd always chosen to suppress these feelings with food; that's how I had been sabotaging my health for several years. Instead of learning what my emotions were attempting to teach me, I squashed them with food. Our food cravings are a metaphor for the reason behind the stuff we must look at so that we can grow, develop, evolve, and move on in life. It's also what we must teach and pass on to others. Some of us pass on info through writing, speaking, painting, and more. My refusal to hear, see, face, and accept this truth is what brought me back to this point in my life, where I had to let go of an additional 50 pounds that I had been holding on to for the past three years. These 50 pounds showed up in my life over and over again. Why? In numerology 50 is 5, and that translates to major life change.

To me, the most logical question is, "What change must I see, hear, feel, taste, smell, and accept as my truth? What change am I afraid of making today?" The answer is simple: It does not mean that I must go looking for something to change. It's that I must be open and receptive to the change coming my way. Letting go of excess fat means that I'm ready to change, that I no longer need to protect myself from that person, place, or thing that is deep within me and wants to get out. I must let go of my fear of feeling hurt, rejected, and abandoned for doing what is in my best interest. There is no need for guilt when I put myself first. This is the time to let myself loose on this big, beautiful world.

People are always going to come and go in our lives. When they teach us what we need to learn, they will either evolve around us or leave. My fear has always been about losing them. That's what happened as a child: they all eventually left me. Over the years I learned to leave them before they had a chance to leave me, as a way of putting myself first. That's from where my fear of commitment came. I no longer try to protect myself from pain—in fact, I welcome it when it happens, because sometimes getting hurt is part of the learning process. Let me make it abundantly clear that I don't *want* to be hurt. The point I am making is that when it happens, I don't run away from it; instead I stay and face it head-on. When needed I do take the time to look at how I'm feeling as events are unfolding around me, and then I address it in that moment. Earlier I talked about the fact that I used food as a tool to cover up and suppress my thoughts, feelings, and emotions. Why is that? Despite knowing how dangerous it is, I still did it. What was I afraid of consciously being aware of? It was partly out of habit as well as a fear of facing my truth and protecting myself from being hurt. My binging was more of a crutch than anything else. Early in my life I'd learned that if I wanted the pain and loneliness to go away, all I had to do was eat. I started with chewing gum and then switched to potato chips and other sweet and crunchy foods. I needed to protect myself from getting hurt, and I used food.

Today I don't need to protect myself, because over the years I've learned how to deal with painful and hurtful situations. When I face all challenges head-on, there is no need to overindulge in food. I've also learned that eating healthy means I'm putting myself first; I'm listening to my body and doing what I love, feel passionate about, and have fun doing. I'm where I want to be.

When I take the time to show myself love, not only do I feel amazing, but I also attract a lot more happy, fun-loving people who always listen to and respect my wishes. When I tell them I need time to rest, they say okay and then check on me in a few days. Setting boundaries and enforcing them leads to more love and respect from all around me.

Guilt and Obligation

Over the years I've been told many times that I must be selfish in order to be successful. People said that without selfishness, I would be taken advantage of and would be walked on. This got me thinking about the types of people with whom I surrounded myself. I concluded that despite having a lot of well-intended, loving friends, their demands on my time could sometimes overwhelm me. Shortly after this realization, I shared it with Patricia, a close friend, and to my surprise she felt the same way. Despite having a group of amazing women as friends, Patricia sometimes felt surrounded by a group of energy vampires. Patricia believed some of them were part of her life because she felt obligated. When she was new to the area, they introduced her to other people, places, and events;

as a result, she felt that she owed them. Knowing Patricia's background, I could clearly see that she had replaced her family with friends, with the same result. With her family, Patricia felt that they had clothed and fed her as a child, and so she must repay them for their kindness. Today, Patricia is still friends with people who take far more than they can give her.

In some ways I can relate to Patricia's story. It all goes back to what I learned from my mom, which is that when someone does something nice for you, then you owe them. The question is, how long before that person is repaid? How much is enough? How will you know when to make the last payment for services rendered?

I have come to understand that people enter our lives for a reason, which is to teach us something. You may have helped me when I needed it, but that does not mean that I owe you. You helped me when I needed help because you wanted to do something nice, but I don't owe you a thing. Looking back, one friend in particular invited me over for Thanksgiving dinner because I was away from my family. I was looking forward to a nice, quiet day alone, so I declined her invitation. So she told me she would no longer be my friend if I didn't come, so I went. I had an okay time, but then I felt forced to go to her home for all holidays.

I realize that these people are wonderful and amazing people who are only trying to do something nice for me. However, that's their interpretation of what I need. It's on me to say no thanks, move on, and not give in to emotional blackmail. I know what's best for me, and I must stick to doing only what feels right for me in that moment.

It's interesting because several years ago I was watching Reverend T. D. Jakes on a televised sermon. He said, "If you are the smartest one in your group of friends, then you need new friends." That struck a chord with me. It's not that I'm smarter than my friends, even though I *am* pretty smart; it's that I'm the one they all turn to with their problems. Although I love helping others, it can be overwhelming when I am a problem solver all day at work and come home to do even more for friends. I sometimes feel that I'm always working without a break. I need to have some fun, but instead I always end up talking about others' issues. I feel that I must put my own needs on hold so that I can help others—at the expense of my personal health. I don't have control over my weight because I consistently put my own feelings and desires on the back burner and use food to punish myself for doing so. My overweight body is a constant reminder that I'm holding on to something that must be set free. It's about letting go of unrealistic expectations and goals for myself and embracing my truth.

My eating is primarily out of control in the evening because it is family time when I'm alone. I have a terrific family with whom I have very little in common. When I'm with them, I find that I give more than I receive. Despite the fact that I care for them very much and only want the best for them, I'm only in touch with them out of obligation. In fact, I have to psych myself up when I have to reach out to them. I know it's not their fault; however, I always feel drained after each visit. It's not only them; I also have friends who drain my energy. So what's the lesson? Why do I continue to attract energy vampires? Is it because I am one myself? No. They are simply reminding me of what I need to maintain a strong, lean, and healthy body. I push them away not because of anything they are doing or saying; it's because I'm resisting the lesson they are teaching me. My energy is drained because I'm putting tons of energy into not wanting to see, hear, know, or accept the message. In other words, I'm blaming the messenger for the message.

It was very clear that just like Patricia, I was substituting friends for my family. That was very interesting to me because I'd moved 3000 miles to get away from the obligations, only to find myself in the same situation with my friends, who I now refer to as Frielients—that's the combination of friend and client—and sometimes the relationship is unclear. They are people I help hours on end but without charging a fee.

I was in the same situation. They were different places and faces, but it was the same situation. If I had any question as to whose issue it was, all I had to do was find the common thread, which was me. You know the old saying that you can't run away from your problems, because no matter where you go, there they are? These Frielients were just the people to teach me a lesson: I needed to let go of my guilt complex. These situations reminded me to look at what I was doing to myself. The energy I was putting into these relationships should and must be redirected into my true love, Healthea Solutions Weight Management Inc. I don't want to hurt them; however, in the end, being honest with them and with myself will help us both.

My top reason for beating myself up with food is the direct result of trying to be there for everyone except myself. It's taking yet another phone call from a Frielient instead of taking the time I need to rest after a long day. It's turning to food because I feel angry for helping others when I need help myself, and I feel guilty when I ignore their call. Sometimes I find myself between a rock and a hard place, and I turn to food to soothe myself.

How have these experiences affected my weight and overall health? I was afraid to ask for help because I didn't want to owe anyone, so I suffered in silence. I suppressed the stress of having to keep them in my life, so I turned to food. Food was the tool I used to cover up and suppress my true feelings so that

I could be there for them. It's also how I chose to punish myself for putting their needs ahead of my own.

Some people look at being a little selfish as a bad thing. If you are in this group, then try replacing selfishness with self-nurturing. In fact, that's exactly what it is: putting yourself first. By taking care of your physical, mental, and emotional health, you will find that you will have more energy to help others. We must balance time with others and time for the self by doing our best to help all in need—when it's appropriate. If it is inconvenient, then we must let them know it's not a good time. We all have friends or family members who are always in conflict about something. When they call, answer and do your best to help them. If you don't want to call them, then don't call, and don't feel guilt or obligation. At some point these people must learn to stand on their own two feet. Guilt-free living is taking care of yourself, which includes and is not limited to eating healthy, getting enough sleep, and exercising. It's taking time for yourself and doing what you love. It's making sure you are living a balanced life free of guilt and obligation.

Optimal health starts at the grocery store, where we are making the decision of whether or not to eat healthy. When we make healthy food choices, then we will be mentally, emotionally, and physically able to handle whatever challenges come our way. When we are feeling good about ourselves, then we will not allow others to take advantage of our good and giving nature. It all starts with us loving and respecting ourselves; others will follow. When we set and enforce strict boundary guidelines of what we will tolerate from our friends and family, the ones who love us will respect them. On the other hand, those who are only out to get what they want regardless of who it hurts will simply move on to someone else. We must prepare ourselves for that possibility, and we must be okay with it. They are not rejecting us; they simply realize that they can't take advantage of us, so they are moving on to someone else they can manipulate.

Have you noticed that specific people come into our lives at a specific time to teach us a specific lesson? At times we experience anger, resentment, or frustration at certain people because we resist this learning. We resist because we are afraid to change that which we know, out of fear of the unknown. I find that they are usually the people I don't like—they are here to showcase my negative behaviours. It's hard to see it in myself, but it's very noticeable in others. On the other hand, the behaviours I like in others are the behaviours I aspire to have. I recently had a conversation with a very good friend who proved this point. She told me that there were three women in her life that she wished would go away. I was surprised because she was a very happy-go-lucky person who got along with everyone. When I asked her what these women had done to evoke that feeling within her, my friend (whom I will call Maxine) answered as follows. With the first woman, Maxine mentioned she was tired of being this woman's councilor. "She is constantly calling and complaining about how unhappy she is in all areas of life. She is never happy for more than five minutes." Maxine told me she did not want to see or talk to her anymore because the woman brought her down, and *Maxine just wanted to have fun.*

Maxine did not want to see the second and third women because they didn't seem to have anything in common anymore, and she *just wanted to have fun.* I then challenged Maxine's opinion of these women by asking a few questions. In the end, Maxine realized that what she was saying about these amazing women was what she actually felt about herself. Maxine was sick and tired about complaining of her lack of happiness in her own life. She realized that despite the fact that she enjoyed her life for the most part, she was simply settling for what was, instead of fighting for what she really wanted. These women were a reflection of how she really felt about herself. At that time Maxine was not ready to face her unhappiness, and that was why she was ready to end these friendships.

Another example of teachers showing up when we need them most happened to me a few years ago. The neighbouring store owner called me and asked if I could give her a hand, because she was short staffed. It was only a few blocks away, so I agreed. When I arrived for my shift, the sales associate who was working with me was very rude to me. I brushed it off and tried to make small talk, to no avail. Finally after a couple of hours I asked her, "Considering the fact you don't know me, why do you dislike me so much?" This sales associate then denied her actions toward me. Interesting enough, immediately after that she was very nice, warm, and friendly toward me.

In this case she was not aware of her actions until I pointed them out. It was not the people, place, or situation with which she had a problem. It was the fact that she didn't like where she was in life and what she was doing. Left unchecked, these feelings can lead to being overweight, to addiction, and even to deep depression.

When it comes to people entering and exiting my life, I've come to understand that with all that I have gone through over the years, it had to have been that way so that I would appreciate all that I have and where I am today. When people show up telling us something about ourselves, if we accept this fact, then they move on. When we don't, then sometimes they stick around; however, it's more likely someone else shows up with the same message but more intensified.

For example, let's say each time you get off the phone with

a loved one, you head straight to the refrigerator even though you are not hungry. You might not have made this connection, but you do know your pants are getting tighter, so you go out and buy new ones. Then one day you meet a new friend, and all you seem to do is talk about her failed relationships. After a few weeks you decide that this person is just like your family members, always nagging you that you don't call enough, so you drop her like a hot potato. Now you find yourself sitting on the coach, watching TV, and eating day after day.

A year later you go in for your annual check-up, and the doctor tells you that you have gained 50 pounds over the past year. You start to look at what, when, and where you were eating. Then the light bulb goes off: you finally understand that you were cutting yourself off from people, and that's why you were turning to food—or was it? That was only part of the answer. The second part happened when you were having a conversation with a stranger. You realized that you were protecting yourself from getting hurt. Throughout your childhood, people were constantly coming into your life and leaving. You have a huge heart and used to love fully. Then when people left, you would have to put the pieces back together. You don't call family members regularly, and you keep your friends at a safe distance because you are afraid of being hurt again. You are afraid that if you allow them to get too close, then when they leave, you might not be able to put yourself back together again.

When we don't want to accept the message that's being delivered, we blame the messenger instead of accepting it with love. In the words of Shakespeare, "To thine own self be true." There are numerous reasons for us to overindulge with food in an attempt to make ourselves feel better. However, the core of it is this simple statement: It's about us being angry at ourselves for being where we don't want to be, doing what we don't want to, and being with people we don't care to be around in that particular moment. It does not mean that you don't love them; it's simply that there is something else you need to do, or someone else you must seek out, or there is somewhere else you need to be in that moment. Knowing your truth will allow you to leave without feeling guilty or obligated to stay any longer than you feel appropriate.

So then why do we continue to be in these relationships when they're sucking the light out of us? It's because we do not want to hurt or let down our friends, family members, or coworkers. We want to be liked and accepted by them, so we suffer in silence. Knowing this, how can we change our way of thinking? We have to be brutally honest with ourselves and put ourselves first. They are our teachers, showing us that we must take better care of ourselves without feeling guilty or obligated to be there for them.

Sometimes the message is twofold. The lesson is teaching us gratitude for who we are, what we do have, and where we are in life today. They are reminding us that all challenges are a gift, and we can discover who we really are at a deeper spiritual level! I went through a period of about three years saying that I found my friends boring. It was not them I was bored with—I was bored with myself. At the time I found that I was doing the same things day in and day out, and I was sick of it. It was much easier to blame them until I took a break from them and travelled deep within myself. Then and only then did I realize I was not living the life I was here to live, and that's why I was attracting all these energy vampires.

Taking time for myself got me back on the right track. Once I came to this realization, my obsessive food craving went away. My inner voice said, "Althea, you just need to stop worrying. Just be. Trust that all is well. You will get to where you need to be at the appointed time. Simply be in the moment, and good things will happen."

The reason I felt I was living someone else's life was because I was living a lie. Professionally speaking, I was in retail, a place where I did not want to be, and I was listening to people haggle over prices. They irritated me because I didn't understand them—or should I say, they were showing me that I really didn't understand myself. Why did I do the things I did and said? The fact that they were constantly asking me what the price was when it was right there on the tag bothered me. I was constantly asking myself why they were so cheap.

Taking time for myself allowed me to see the big picture. In fact, they were asking me to look closely at what my job was costing me. I had to take a closer look at what was in front of me. All I had to do was open my eyes, and I would see the truth of how I'd been treating myself.

Guilt and obligation can make us fat if we let them. When we are where we don't want to be and are doing what we don't to do, we tend to turn to food for support. Why do we choose to suffer in silence instead of speaking our truth? We must speak up and let others know that we are not interested. If they are hurt, then it's on them, not us; they can choose to be offended or accept the information in the spirit that it was intended. The thing to remember is that it's us or them. Yes, we must help all who need our help, but charity begins at home. If these energy vampires are to be in our lives, then it must be mutually beneficial to both of us. If they are to be there permanently, then we would not feel the way we do today. Things that are meant to be are easy.

We must create room to study, learn, grow, and develop as individuals so that we can help others when needed. We must take responsibility for our own healing and health. I know it's tempting to blame others for being pains in our asses, but we need to set boundaries with them. They are happy with the way things are because they are getting their needs met, and we are not. It's about getting our needs met mentally, emotionally, and physically. When we do, we are happy and eat healthy foods to nourish our bodies. When our needs are not met, we turn to food to self-medicate, thus avoiding our pain of not being fed appropriately.

Emotional Connection

Over the years I've learned that when I eat small, healthy meals, I tend to have lots of energy, a clear mind, and a happy spirit; I want to exercise, write, and do the right thing to maintain my healthy body. I also have a clear mind and a happy spirit. So why don't I do so consistently? It's because sometimes I want to avoid feeling hurt.

When all is well in our lives, then for optimal health we eat healthy foods for our constitutions, we engage in fun physical exercises, and we meditate daily. However, eating the right foods consistently and exercising is easier said than done. In my life today I eat too much dairy, wheat, and sugar when I'm stressed out; I'm beating myself up for being where I don't want to be. Why? Because it's easier to bury my desire within than to face it.

Like it or not, everything we eat affects our health, whether negatively or positively. I believe that most of us know what to eat, but we don't. Why is that? There are thousands if not millions of books out there telling us how to lose weight. I have tried several of them myself. So why is our weight still not where we want it to be? It's because it's not the weight—it's what the weight symbolizes. Our bodies are a classroom to teach us lessons that we can't learn any other way. My million-dollar question is, "Body, what message do you have for me today?"

To start, the majority of my excess weight is in my abdominal area—right in front of me, where I am forced to deal with it in this lifetime. What does the abdomen symbolize to me? It's the way I take in, digest, and eliminate things. My body is telling me I'm taking on too much and leaving little time for rest. Taking on too much in a short period leaves me with very little time to digest and analyze the information I'm getting. There's not enough time to formalize and execute a plan. It's telling me to stop, listen, and focus on my goals, instead of standing in my own way. The most important question to overweight people is that with all we know about nutrition and weight loss, why do we continue to binge on junk food and eat late at night? It's important to look at the time of day you are most likely to turn to food for comfort. What's happening around you? What are you longing for? In that moment, what's missing in your life? In my case the answer was that I was not living for myself; I was too busy taking care of everyone else. When one of my life centres is out of balance, I binge. It's interesting because I was also eating out of frustration of not living on purpose. However, part of that was being prepared for my role. I had to take better care of myself so that I could be there for others without guilt. It's like when the flight attendants state that in case of emergency, one should put on one's own mask first. I must do the same. The question then becomes how? The answer is that I must physically put it into my schedule each and every day, and I must stick to the program no matter what challenges appear. In fact, by taking time out for me, I find that I can spot the answer to problems much sooner.

For many years I knew that retail management was not

my dream, and yet I stayed despite feeling trapped in the wrong profession. By following the signs of the universe, I realized that I had to remain in retail for now. The million-dollar question was how could I lose 50 pounds while working in retail—and keep it off permanently? It was very simple: I must take scheduled time each day to study, write, and teach weight management to women. I was aware that I had to make a living; however, it did not mean that I had to put all my time and energy into it. I must do the best job I was being paid to do and at the same time focus on where I wanted to go. By knowing where I was today, I could accept the fact that this was a temporary situation and focus on where I was going. I gave thanks for today and moved on to tomorrow.

I believe that maintaining a healthy weight is living on purpose. With that said, I do know my life's purpose is to help women manage their weight by releasing negative, toxic energy stores in their fatty tissues. Along with that, I must take time out for me each and every day. It takes a lot of energy to help, and I must replenish my energy through proper nutritional intake, physical exercise, meditation, and rest. It's about helping women who are in need of my support.

I attract the type of people I do so that I can put my listening skills into practice. I am a great coach who is suppressing her own skill. I have been blessed with the ability to hear the truth in their voices and see the pain in the faces of these women. All I have to do is listen and give my opinion as to what's happening to them.

I abuse my body with excessive consumption of harmful foods because I have not achieved my person goals in the area of health accomplishments. I am angry and frustrated at the speed at which I am progressing in this area. I have put everything else on the line for them. The thing is, it does not matter how much I want to achieve with them, they will not happen until it's the right time and place.

The choice is mine. I can continue to push on a closed door, or I can patiently wait for it to open when it's right. "What you resist persists." By continually pushing my own agenda before the time is right, I only cause more personal pain. I then push away the three things I want most by eating and gaining weight, by spending and putting myself into more debt, and by resisting moving on and up in retail. Its time I let go and trust the universe's plan for me. It's time I start living in the moment. I should be present with my life as it's unfolding in the moment. I should stop pressuring myself to do something that's not meant to be today.

My relationship with food—what is it all about? I've been under the impression that it's all resolved around my anger at myself. Another part of that anger is a result of extreme anger at all the grown-ups who were supposed to be there for me but were not; they abandoned me night after night. They were not there for me when I was sad and needed comforting. They were not there to answer my questions when I was curious. These people are Mom, Mama, and my uncles, as well as the father I never knew.

It all started when I was a child in Jamaica, and I was left alone a lot of the time. The way my mother and grandmother showed me love was by making sure I had enough to eat, and as a result I've carried on the tradition.

What if I were to tell you that it's not entirely accurate? Another reason I eat food in the evening is that I have not eaten enough during the day, and as a result I start grazing. During the day my mind is occupied with work and other thoughts. However, in the evening my mind is free to think about food. When people let me down, I rationalize it, forgive them, and turn to food to beat up myself. I blame myself for others abandoning me and turning me down. I blame myself by telling myself I am not good enough, that I deserve to be taken advantage of.

Looking back, I was denied what I believed I deserved, so I turned to food because I blamed myself for causing the outcome. I was fat because I was angry. I took on the blame instead of placing it on the person to whom it belonged. Instead of getting angry with others for disappointing me, I turned on myself. This was where it started, and all the other disappointments are measured by these events, or should I say standards. When someone says no to me, I traumatize myself. The solution to my food compulsion is coming to terms with my feelings in the moment. I can choose to blame others, or I can choose to accept what is, forgive, and move on with my life. This is healthy being and thinking.

Here is what I do know for sure. My obsessive thought of food is triggered by my childhood memory of being left alone in the evenings as a child. When Mama was unable to come home to take care of me, she would send food to keep me company until she or one of my uncles could come home. I was always afraid when it got dark, which was the fear of being alone. The food represented companionship. With all that said, how could I change my thinking pattern? Here I was at 47 years old, and I kept replaying this tape over and over again.

Two questions gave me the answer. The first was, "What lesson am I to learn from that experience?" The answer is self-reliance! I am never alone because I always have myself to rely on. During this time of feeling lonely, I must go deep within to find my voice, the message. I'm in this position because that's where I need to be in order to learn and to be exposed to this learning! From a very early age, the consistent message from the universe and everyone around me was that I must take care of me because I know how to. I am enough! I do have enough knowledge about how to take care of my mental, emotional, and physical health. All I need to do is be still long enough to receive this wonderful message. The second question was, "What message can I replace the old tape with?" Keep telling myself that I am enough, that I'm complete, that I'm all that I seek. I should look within for the answers. This fear I'm experiencing in this moment will pass, making way to uncover the beautiful message and enhance my spiritual growth. I've come to understand that feeling abandoned as a child only plays a minor role in my life today. What's causing me more of a problem is being ignored, which is connected to being ignored a great deal as a child. So how and what can I do today to heal this pain, anger, and frustration of being ignored by others? This reminds me of a situation that happened when I was in high school. I was in sewing class, attempting to make a dress. I cut out the pattern and was sewing it. This is a class in which I excelled; I loved it, and it came very easy to me. On this particular day, for some reason I was having difficulty following the directions of the pattern, so I put my hand up, signalling for Mrs. Gabriel to come over and assist me.

I did that for about 15 minutes, and I knew she saw me; however, she did not come over to help. I then packed up my things and put away the sewing machine. This was an extra class, and I was not getting credit for it, so I decided to leave. I went over to Mrs. Gabriel and told her that I was leaving because I couldn't seem to focus. Then to my surprise she said, "I did not come over because I wanted you to figure it out on your own. You are a very smart girl, and I have confidence in you." I left the classroom, stunned.

Am I being ignored by others because they believe that

I can figure it out on my own? I see a theme here; can you? Being left alone or ignored sucks, but it does not mean that one is not loved or wanted. Sometimes people are not there for us because they have faith and confidence in us and in our ability to entertain ourselves. We can figure out how to get our needs met when we put our minds to it.

As human beings we are designed to avoid pain and seek pleasure. In order to experience happiness, I participate in the overconsumption of unhealthy foods despite being aware of the consequences to my health. What I've come to understand is that despite the pain, I must let things happen in the moment so that I can experience, learn, and develop as a well-rounded spiritual being. I need to be still long enough to understand the learning. It will happen one way or the other. Stop taking thing so personally and instead accept the message being delivered. You are a brilliant mind with free will. You can do it once you put your mind to it. In fact, it's more gratifying when you do it yourself. You can choose to be angry at others for not being there for you, or you can choose to be happy with yourself and your abilities.

Regardless of how old you are and how many people you know, there will be many times when you will have to experience being home all alone, and you will experience all the emotions that go with it. You can play the victim game, the "poor me" card, or you can learn and grow. I believe excessive weight gain symbolizes a rejection of self. It's a clear indication that our true wants, needs, and desires are being unfulfiled. Over the years while working with numerous women, I found that there are three types of overweight women. The first group is overweight because of food. To manage their weight, all they have to do is watch what they eat, as well as when and how. They should look at food sensitivities as well.

Elizabeth Hasselbeck, former cohost on *The View,* fits into this category. Once she figured out that she had celiac disease, her health issues went away. This group makes up 10 percent of people.

The second group has issues with weight because of unresolved emotions. The best way to address the problem is to visit a certified health-care professional for assistance in identifying and dealing with these emotions. This group is also 10 percent of the overweight population.

The third group, with the remaining 80 percent, is a very complicated group that involves both of the first two. One day it's because of what they eat, and the next day they are eating our emotions. They are always going back and forth, sometimes hour by hour.

Some of us are overweight because of a paralyzing emotion. In this situation, I believe all afflictions and diseases are a direct result of our unresolved emotions. Ask yourself, 'What feelings and emotions am I holding on to? What am I afraid to see, hear, know, feel, smell, and believe about my life? What am I running away from? Why am I afraid to live a strong, lean, healthy, and balanced life? Why am I afraid of being loving and compassionate toward myself? Why am I willing to be there for others in their times of need, regardless of how inconvenient it is for me? Why do I put my own well-being on hold?"

By now I've made it very clear that I believe being overweight is a clear indication that one is hiding or suppressing something within one's physical body. In most cases we are not aware of what we are doing to ourselves; we simply know we are gaining weight despite eating healthy and exercising regularly.

In my case, it's because of anger. I was angry because despite my desire to work as a full-time weight management coach, I was still in retail. I wanted more than just a few clients a month—I wanted to help millions, not thousands of women. I was angry at the fact that I was not as successful as I wanted to be.

I believe that subconsciously, I expected to be rejected by potential clients. As I thought, so I manifested. It's interesting because on January 1, 2010, I wrote in my journal that to have everything I dreamed of, all I had to do was reach my goal weight and keep it for six months. Today I am approximately 20 pounds heavier; I still believe this today. I want to make it abundantly clear that it's not about losing weight, or being rich, or being self-employed. It's about embracing all that I am today without fear of losing or being abandoned.

Knowing all this, what is my next move? How do I reach my goal weight and stop hurting my beautiful body? In the end it's my choice. I can choose to give my body energy, or I can rob it of vital nutrients. I must become who I'm meant to be today, or I can blame others for where I am in life. In the end I choose to be open and receptive to my personal thoughts, feelings, and beliefs about myself. Being the kind of person I am born to be involves facing my emotions head-on. For those of us hiding our emotions, we must remember the root cause of all illnesses and afflictions are unexpressed emotions! Express these hidden emotions, and your condition will be healed. What are your emotional wounds? What makes you happy or sad? Part of dealing with your emotions is naming your feelings. Not too long ago, I was at a marketing seminar. There were nine experts speaking on topics ranging from how to get published, to how to start a blog, to all the different types of social media. Halfway through the second day, I found myself in a position where, despite learning lots, I was thinking of eating junk food. Why was that? I started to ask myself what I was trying to cover up and suppress. What was

I afraid of? What was so scary that I was choosing to break my personal commitment to myself to lose 20 pounds? I then realized that I was experiencing information overload. I was feeling overwhelmed with all the information I was getting.

Once I identified that I was feeling overwhelmed, and that was why I was thinking of food, the craving went away and I was able to focus on the speaker. The next obvious question was what kind of relief was I getting from food, and what could I substitute it with? I was regressing to my childhood, where food was what we used to make ourselves feel better instead of facing what was happening in the moment. I did not know what to do, so I fell back on food.

This incident caused me to see that this is a pattern for me. When I'm feeling overwhelmed with all that's happening within and outside of me, I turn to food for comfort. Being overwhelmed means that there is so much to do, and I feel very confused as to what to do next. What direction is best for me? What I've realized over the years in retail management is to simply make a list of everything I want to get done and prioritize it, and I will instantly feel better because I'm clear on where I'm going. So is that my Healthea Solution to maintaining my weight? That's definitely part of the equation.

Whether or not you want to admit it, we all have emotional baggage. There are thoughts feelings and behaviours we hold on to based on our experiences in life. For example, when I'm feeling rejected, it's because of one or two reasons: it's because I'm rejecting myself, or it's because I'm rejecting the message. They are indeed a mirror, reflecting back to me my own behaviour. To put it another way, when I feel hurt by others who ignore me or pretend not to see or hear me it's residue from my childhood. When I'm feeling left out, my mind goes back to that 6-year-old little girl in Jamaica, after Papa died.

At this point in my life, for the most part I recognize my feelings in an instant and correct them right then and there. However, there are times when I have an overwhelming day or am dealing with a particular situation that is insurmountable. I then take it out on the person or group that is reminding me of my past pain and hurt. I do so by deliberately withdrawing from the situation, ignoring their presence, and judging them and thinking that I'm better than them. I think that they're not okay the way they are. I then become so disgusted with myself that I turn to food to feel better.

I'm a highly excitable, emotional person who sometimes uses food as a tool to ground myself. I attempt to stay grounded long enough to let it out and let it go. I've learned that I attract others who push my buttons so that I can see what emotional baggage is weighting me down, and then I can change it.

If you are an angry person, then that's who you attract. Other angry people are here to show you who you are and what you've been suppressing. You must acknowledge this and let it out, let it go, and let it be. When I'm feeling triggered by others, I take a few minutes to ask myself a few questions: "Why am I getting this information at this point? What am I experiencing at this moment?" Once you master this technique, it only takes seconds within the moment to become untriggered. With practice you will get so good that no one will have a clue that you were triggered. Once you are healed, then that person will move on to someone else.

People who are triggers are telling me that I must get comfortable and understand what it's like to be alone, because once I'm in a loving, romantic relationship, I will do what it takes to nurture and grow it. I need to remember my childhood and all those nights I was left alone. The thing is that there is a good chance it will happen again. I hope it doesn't, but if it does, I know it's just a test to see how I will react. Will I dry my tears and move on to the next relationship, or will I bury my feelings? It's about facing my feelings head-on.

To be healthy in mind and body, we must understand and then let go of the past so that we can embrace the future. Everything that has happened to us thus far in life is not an accident. No matter how devastating it was, it taught us something and made us a stronger and better person.

When I'm feeling ignored, it's usually because I'm ignoring my own needs and desires. These people are telling me to stop putting the needs of others ahead of my own. I must focus on where I want to be. It's time for me to be selfish and take care of myself first. The triggers are reminding me that I'm worth being first on my list.

The liver is the seat of our emotions. One time I had been experiencing bad nausea for a few days, which puzzled me. I expressed my concern to my assistant, who asked me if I was pregnant. I told her I was post-menopausal, which meant that ship had sailed. I then said to myself, "It's a buildup of excess toxins in my liver, which is being disturbed each time I eat unhealthy foods." I decided to complete a liver cleanse on Saturday and Sunday. Throughout the afternoon I realized that despite not being 100 percent, I felt much better. It made me realize that the pain always goes away once I face the truth.

Today I'm reminded of how complex we are as human beings in thoughts, feelings, and beliefs. To be a well-rounded individual, I feel I must have numerous interests. For me, this includes but is not limited to reading, writing, and teaching weight management, spirituality, symbolism, and power walking. What all this comes down to is that I thoroughly enjoy the meaning behind human behaviours. I'm fascinated by why we do the things we do, make the decisions we do, and surround ourselves with certain people. What lesson are we to learn from them, and what message are we to deliver to them?

Stress Meter

Just like everything we eat affects our health, everything we feel also contributes to our physical health. When we are feeling stressed—be it mentally, emotionally, or physically—there is a price to pay if we are not careful. In certain situations stress can help us because it's short-term, which we can then channel into a positive outcome.

What you have to be concerned about is chronic stress. What's the biggest stressor in your life today? For me, the biggest stress throughout my adulthood has been my retail job. Here is an example. It was my day off, and I had just finished my dental appointment. I was walking to the library, which was only two blocks away, when I received a call from my assistant telling me that my boss had called and said it was mandatory for all store managers to be on the conference call at 1:00 p.m. The voice mail said if the store manager was off, then the person picking up the message must call her and tell her. Even though it was only 10:00 a.m. and the call was at 1:00 p.m., I decided not to take the call. I called her and told her I already had plans that couldn't be changed, because I was on my way for this appointment. If she did not want my assistant to take it, I would get the information from one of the managers later.

After getting the notes from one of the managers who was on the call, I was not surprised that there was nothing of great importance on the call. All that was discussed was how to improve business on the week, and we are already ahead of projections. She also discussed what to expect from the regional manager's meeting in six days.

I managed a very busy and fast-paced store, and I hated every minute of it. On my day off I sometimes found it hard to turn it off. Being told to interrupt my day off to take a conference call caused me more stress. When I was stressed, I turned to food to suppress my anger at myself for sticking with this profession. The high-calorie, processed foods served as a source of comfort for me, but they are a double-edged sword. On one hand they provided the emotional release I craved, and on the other hand they derailed my health.

People ask me all the time, "What is stress?" Stress is experiencing mental, emotional, or physical tension, strain, or distress. The next logical question is, "What causes stress?" There are two types of stress. The first is external stressors, ranging from not being able to find the keys, heavy traffic, an overbearing boss, or the constant social stresses of life (dealing with people's tempers, aggression, and anger). Major events such as losing a job, being passed over for a promotion, having a new baby, or experiencing a death in the family are also included. We generate most of this stress ourselves. We make poor lifestyle choices, we have stressful personality traits, we are hard on ourselves, and we fall into unproductive mind traps.

The second type is internal stressors, which include negative self-talk ("I am stupid"), living an unhealthy life (smoking, excessive coffee, staying up late and rising early), mental traps ("Now that I lost 25 pounds, my life will be perfect." "My boss is not smiling, so he must hate my report"), and personality blues (working too much and too hard). It also includes the following chemical stresses.

Caffeine

- Coffee is a stimulant drug that triggers a stress response in your body.
- It draws the B vitamins out of the body, which are needed to reduce stress and support the adrenal glands.
- After the initial pick-up, you have an energy drop.
- The elimination of caffeine from your diet will result in better sleep, calmer nerves, more energy, fewer muscle aches, less heartburn, and fewer headaches.

Alcohol

- Too much alcohol increases stress because it interferes with healthy, natural sleep.
- Use in moderation.

Nicotine

- The toxins in smoke raise the heart rate and stress the entire body, from the brain to the immune system.

Diet High in Starch and Sugar

Sugar is more of a tranquilizer than an energy supply. The body copes with a sugar rush by secreting insulin, which promptly cuts the amount of sugar in the blood. In terms of stress management, sugar gives you a quick burst of energy followed by a low-energy feeling because of the upset balance of your blood sugar level; this upset can then bring on the stress attractor hyperglycaemia.

If you suffer from low blood sugar, you are more vulnerable to stress, partly because you are feeling tired all the time and partly because hyperglycaemia slows down thinking and concentration.

How does stress affect weight management? If you are overweight, and if you have tried numerous diets only to regain the weight, then chances are you are unable to maintain your ideal weight due to elevated levels of cortisol brought on by chronic stress. Cortisol is the primary hormone of stress and is the body's anti-inflammatory chemical. It can affect nearly every system in our body. The following are symptoms associated with cortisol imbalance:

- cravings for salt, sugar, and carbohydrates
- mood swings and irritability
- fluctuation in energy levels throughout the day
- feeling that the daily demands of life are overwhelming
- insomnia—usually the first indication of cortisol imbalance. Falling asleep is not a problem, but by 2:00 or 3:00 a.m. one is wide awake for 30 minutes or longer. Disturbed sleeping patterns are brought on by a particularly worrisome or stressful situation.

The hormonal system is a negative feedback loop: it produces specific chemicals to initiate specific reactions, and when they are raised to a level of overabundance, the system triggers a mechanism to turn it off. This is homeostasis, and it is largely regulated by the automatic nervous system.

The orchestration of human stress response resides in the automatic nervous system, which is divided into the sympathetic and parasympathetic branches. The automatic nervous system controls our breathing, digestion, blood pressure, blinking, and thinking. The sympathetic automatic nervous system gets things going and is activity oriented. The body has sympathetic nerve endings on almost every organ, muscle, and blood vessel to facilitate its functions. The adrenal glands, located superior to our kidneys, also secrete the hormones epinephrine and norepinephrine to stimulate the sympathetic system in times of stress. On the other end of the neurological spectrum is the parasympathetic branch, which puts the brakes on the system.

The role of the sympathetic system is to pump out hormones that increase heart rate, respiration, blood pressure, and muscle strength for exercise, or for responding to physical danger. Then the parasympathetic system counter-balances the sympathetic activity to restore calm, promote relaxation, and facilitate digestive function, energy storage, and tissue repair and growth when the danger has passed.

As the sympathetic system becomes engaged in the stress response, be it physiological or psychological, a cascade of hormonal events occurs. The body cannot differentiate between physical and psychological stressors, and that's where the limbic system comes in. The limbic system includes the hippocampus, the thalamus, the hypothalamus, the pituitary gland, and the thalamus. The thalamus receives all incoming information and dispatches it to the hippocampus. Upon initiation of the stress response, the hypothalamus releases corticotropin-releasing factor (CRF), and the pituitary gland releases adrenocorticotropin (ACTH), which causes the adrenal glands to secrete cortisol. Once the stress is resolved, the cortisol circulates back to the hypothalamus, and the system shuts down. With chronic or repetitive stress, however, the hypothalamus can become desensitized to cortisol and is unable to stop the pituitary gland from signalling the adrenal glands to keep secreting cortisol. This is like the thermostat in your home malfunctioning so that it does not know when it is hot enough, and therefore it does not turn off the furnace.

Elevated levels of cortisol are dangerous because during a stress response, the body will not be engaged in the growth or repair of tissues, and it suppresses the immune system.

The Weight of Moving

Over the years I've moved many times for various reasons, both personal and professional. With each move I put on weight. Why? At the time I was not sure, and it took many years to finally figure it out. In this case, putting on weight was not about the past but about the present. It was about me moving to a place I didn't want to be and feeling that I didn't have a choice.

Am I saying that I put weight on because I was lacking choice? In part, yes! I was being a good soldier and went in the direction I was instructed to go. In most cases I knew it was the wrong direction to take; however, I consumed unhealthy foods to suppress that voice from within. As a result of my voice not being heard, my body had no choice but to show me what I was doing to myself.

One such example is when I moved from Vancouver to Victoria. It started when a very close friend of mine asked me to support her in the Victoria marathon. The night before the race, I could not sleep. I tried meditation and music, but it did not help. Finally I fell asleep around 4:00 a.m., only to awake soon after. Immediately I felt this strong pull to move there. I thought about it and thought it was crazy, so I decided to keep it to myself. A few hours later my friend and I were walking to the race when out of nowhere I told her that I'd decided to move to Victoria and why.

Immediately after, I felt very excited. The following Monday I chickened out of telling my boss about my plan, and I came down with a very bad cold. During this time there were two songs I could not stop humming: "The Midnight Train to Georgia" by Gladys Knight and the Pips, and "Sitting on the Dock of the Bay" by Otis Redding.

A few days later, I was helping my boss open up a new

store, and at the end of the shift I finally pulled her aside and told her. To my surprise her response was, "What are you going to do about a job?" I told her I did not know; I simply knew that I had to move there. Her next comment was, "What about Mayfair?" I was shocked. She told me that the store manager's position in that store was open, so I accepted the transfer.

I thought I was moving there permanently, but it did not work out this way. I had a difficult time adjusting to the city. The first sign that this move was temporary was when I was having difficulty focusing on unpacking my belongings. Usually after a big move I unpacked everything and was fully set up within 24 hours. I don't like my things in boxes—they must be where I can see them. That first weekend that I set aside for moving was spent walking around the beautiful city feeling sad without knowing why. My weight increased because I was very uncomfortable where I was, and here I was in a new city hundreds of miles away from my friends, all alone. To ground myself and make myself feel safe and secure, I ate all the wrong foods, and that's why I gained weight with each move.

So why was I constantly moving? I did it to grow, learn, and experience life. In the end I realized that I simply did not want to be there. You may ask, "Why not?" As beautiful a city as it was, I found it to be extremely slow pace. It was exactly what I needed: a place where I could take the time to focus on my goals.

So how can I do the above without gaining weight? At first I view the weight gain as a sign for me to stop moving and settle down in one place, to plant roots in one place. I need to take the excess weight off and keep it off because I believe this excess fat is standing in my way of my growth and development on a spiritual level. I can travel, but I must always come home to my base.

Today I view it as there was a lesson there to be learned. I was in Victoria where the pace was much slower, and I walked everywhere. I needed to be there and focus on my personal health and fitness level.

Moving is very stressful due to all the planning, organizing, and orchestrating, from finding a place to live to the packing and unpacking to getting adjusted in the new place. I followed the emotional roller coaster of weight gain and realized that worrying made me fat. You see, when I'm stressed I worry, and when I am worried I turn to food to cover up, suppress, and calm me down. Knowing this, my question then is, "Why can't you just stop worrying about things over which you have absolutely no control? What is that little voice inside your head saying?" I worry when I'm not sure it's the right thing for me to do. I felt that I had no choice but to move to Victoria; however, I did, and not knowing brought on the worry. In sports they always ask the champions, "If you could talk to the younger you, what advice would you give him?" My advice to the younger me is to focus on the here and now, to enjoy each and every moment, because the ride ahead is wild, and you will wish you have time to rest. So enjoy the here and now in this beautiful period of rest and discovery. Once you have made the decision to do something, stop worrying because what's done is done. Whether good or bad, only time will tell.

Worry causes pain, and pain is resistant of the truth that this is where I'm supposed to be. Choosing not to accept the stages that I am at in this moment, because I don't like the people, place, or thing that's happening in my life today, means I am refusing to grow and refusing to accept the lessons of the universe because I don't like the package it's in or its time frame. It's amazing how I am much happier when I accept events as they happen, and as a result an answer to my question shows up shortly thereafter. For example, I missed the bus because the door I usually exit, which is close to the bus stop, was locked. I then had to take another exit and consequently take a later bus. When I got on the bus and looked at the schedule, I realized that on Sundays the bus leaves at 11:39, not 11:17, meaning I did not have to wait long at Surrey central. My goal is to learn to be present in mind, body, and spirit. Regardless of the potential for pain, I want to experience life as is in each moment. I'm committed to looking at my behaviour and reactions in each given moment in order to understand what it is that I'm suppressing and running away from. One day in a casual conversation with Trang, my personal trainer, I told her that the main reason for my weight gain is that I am angry at myself for not being in my chosen profession as a weight management coach. Then I was watching PBS, and a woman talked about shame. I found it boring, so I turned it off after about 30 minutes. I thought that even though I experience shame sometimes, for the most part none of it applies to my life today. Then today I notice how many time I would say to myself that I "hate" this, that, or the other thing. I then remember the woman saying, "When you use that phrase, it's out of shame." I tied the two together and concluded that I was ashamed of being a store manager. This is where I must be and what I must do, so how can I release this shame now? It's all about showing a little patience. It's not the moving that's making you fat. You are not keeping your word to yourself because you are angry with yourself for not being where you want to be. You are a healer and want to make a comfortable living helping others to heal in mind, body, and spirit. The universe is telling you "not now," and all you heard is no. What you are doing is blaming yourself because you believe "not now" to mean "not ever."

I've concluded that despite all the worry and impatience, I'm still on the right track. One day you will be paid handsomely for your work; simply be patient and believe in your abilities. Accept your gift wholeheartedly. In the meantime, take the opportunity to know yourself better. There are teachers all around you showing you those parts of you that you love and dislike. The point of all this is for you to learn to accept all of your past without judgment. It's about acknowledging and experiencing all parts of the self without being affected negatively or positively.

Why did I continue to sabotage myself for so many years? Recently I had a very interesting conversation with my sister, Aveta. I asked her what was new, and her response was, "You know, same old, same old."

I then responded by saying, "Well, you love the status quo."

She laughed and said yes. Then she went on to tell me that the worst thing that had happened to her over the past five years occurred a couple weeks back, when she went for a bike ride and got a flat tire with no gas station in sight. Then she got lost walking around trying to find one.

I then shared with her that I thrive on change. After the conversation I could not get my statement out of my head. After much thought I realized that on a conscious level that's true; however, on a subconscious level I'm much more like my sister.

I did not realize it until now, but to me status quo means routine. It's the same thing each and every day; you know what to expect from each move you make, and nothing ever changes. I find this boring, uninteresting, and unmotivating—or do I? When I get bored, there is usually some opportunity for me to move. For me, moving is chasing excitement. The thing is that I can find excitement wherever I am. Chasing it taught me that it's within me no matter where I move; all I have to do is let it out.

Looking back, when I'm in one place for a while and resist the need to move, I usually find something else to motivate me, such as writing this book. A few months prior to the start of this writing venture, I came very close to quitting my job, but in the 11th hour I decided to stay. It is one of the best decisions I have ever made.

Moving is not a bad thing. What I'm saying is that you should look at the reason for and frequency in which you move. Ask yourself, "Am I moving toward something, or am I running away from something?" I worked for one company for four years and was in six stores. I went in, made it profitable, and then was asked to do the same in another store. This worked for the company but not for me, because I was not able to put down roots. I was not even able to enjoy my success before moving on to another challenge. I turned to food for comfort because I was lacking the balance of a healthy lifestyle.

Living a healthy lifestyle is a choice we all must consciously make. Healthy living results in a strong, lean, healthy body. It's announcing to the entire world that you do care about the way you look and feel each and every day—not in an egotistical way but instead from a place of love of yourself and humankind. It's learning how to put yourself first so that you will have the energy to help others. With that said, the following pages are full of ideas of balancing your health centre. The first step is living a clean existence.

Clean living is the absence of toxins from the food we eat, the home, career choices, spending habits, relationships, spirituality connectedness, personal growth, and development. It's looking at each area and identifying the toxic thoughts, feelings, and behaviours associated with everyone involve, and then cleaning house. Remember, it's loving to let go of people, places, and situations that no longer make you feel happy, content, and fulfiled. In a way, it's about portion control. We must realize that sometimes in our lives, less is more. Spreading ourselves too thin is detrimental to our health. Toxic living affects every aspect of one's life, including but not limited to: increased hot flashes in menopausal women, interruptions in sleep patterns us, increased anger resentment and frustration of life, excessive weight gain, reduced self-esteem, and increased fatigue. As you can see from the list above, it's more than making us fat. In a nutshell, putting toxic elements into our wonderful bodies, minds, and spirits takes away more then it gives. So why the heck does we continue to do this to ourselves? We *do* know better, so why don't we do better?

Cleaning involves you doing what you love, feel passionate about, and have fun doing. It's being where you want to be and being surrounded by people who encourage mental, emotional, physical, and spiritual stimulation. As a result, you will find that you have everything you have ever dreamed of, which can include but is not limited to these things:

- a successful career
- romance
- happiness
- financial independence
- optimal health
- spiritual and personal awareness
- strong leadership
- greatness
- being more connected with God and the entire universe
- being alive

The three components to health are the balancing of the mind, body, and spirit. To achieve optimal health, all three must be in harmony with each other. You will find that when you are eating lots of vegetables, some protein, and fruits along with a small amount of dairy (substitute) and grains, you are more mentally alert, you are emotionally balanced, your spirit is high, and your body is healthy. You then sleep better and have lots of energy to do everything you enjoy doing. With healthy eating habits, you will find you are more alert and receptive to the signs of the universe.

Why do I want to lose weight? It's not about losing weight—it's about permanent weight management. When I look in the mirror, all I can see are the lies I tell myself, and my anger and fears that I continue to bury in my abdominal cavity. I desperately want to let go of it all, but I continue to give in to my food cravings. I've come to realize that cravings are not necessarily about the need for food as much as they're about needing to be nurtured in a particular part of my life. Food is how the universe is getting my attention.

I now view food cravings as approaching life's situations as lessons designed to awaken and move me forward in life. I am being guided, and all I must do is accept my teachers; they will lead me thought the path of rightfulness. Food craving is a sign reminding me to focus on my health and well-being. I'm looking at all seven life centres, and letting go of all that no longer serves me. Being healthy for me is letting things go without worry or fear of not having it when I need it in the future. I have all I need within me today and always. Being mentally, emotionally, and physically healthy means we are ready for success. We are prepared to live the life we are meant to live. As a result, we only eat to sustain health.

When we are not ready to live the abundant life, we are

here to live, and then temptation always raises its head, be it food, drugs, or any other form of addiction. So what's standing in your way of accepting authentic self? Do you feel that you deserve to live a content, fulfiled, and healthy life? Do you feel that you deserve success and abundance? When you truly believe the answer is yes to these questions, more doors will be opened for you. Which door will you walk through? That's why I say pick one and run with it. Keep moving despite whatever fear you might be experiencing. You must not stand in your own way. Successful weight management is about commitment, about deciding what you want. Commit, water it daily with gratitude of where you are going, and see what happens. Water it with patience and watch it grow. When you truly believe, you will commit and fight for it. Don't hesitate; to commit is to take action, and that equals success.

We have free will to choose the path that's open to us and brings peace or to choose our own ego-based agenda and live an unhappy existence. A good rule of thumb is that if you are going against who you are and what you do, you will be unhappy. When you are being authentic, things that you thought were out of your reach will unexpectedly show up.

It's fair to say my thinking of food when not hungry is my subconscious reaction to a particular memory, block, energy, and vibration. I experience these feelings because there is something that I must face; however, I'm afraid to do so because I'm unable to see the big picture of how it fits into my life. At this point I am unable to see its connection to my goal.

Food cravings are a warning that all is not well, that I'm out of balance in thought. It's a trigger telling me to get in touch with what I'm feeling in that precise moment. The same can be said for being overweight. It's telling us that we are not happy where we are in this instant, that we must focus on what we are feeling, doing, and saying. It's a sign for us to ask, "Is this what I want to be doing? Is this how I want to spend my time? What am I to understand and learn from this person, place, or situation?" Focus on where you want to be doing and with whom, and then water it with patience; the cravings will stop.

My desire to live a balanced life is what fuels me. My greatest desire is to know the real, authentic Althea. It's not that I need to be thin; it's that being thin means I am open to receive and give love to myself and to everyone around me. It's a matter of being free to welcome others into my world, tearing down that protective wall I've built around myself, and knowing the only fear is that which is within me.

I was afraid of what I was experiencing in this moment, so I turned to food to suppress my truth. I've found that simply identifying and accepting how I'm feeling in each moment is all I need to turn away from unhealthy eating patterns. Instead, I embrace my truth and feed myself love and understanding of who I am and the role I play in life. I accept the fact that it's okay to be me. I've come to understand that to be truly happy, I must accept the fact that I am the source of all my pain and unhappiness in my life. My pain is a result of the type of people I invite into my personal life. Since I was a child, I've always attracted the wounded, and then I felt that I had no choice because most of the wounded were family members in charge of my care, health, and well-being. Today I'm a grown-up, and as such I have the right to say, "Stop. Enough is enough."

For my own mental health and well-being, I have to say what I will do and won't do for them without feeling guilty. In order to be happy, content, and fulfiled, I had to say goodbye to negative people in my personal life and embrace positive ones. I love helping people who are in emotional pain; however, in order to live a strong, lean, and healthy life, I must keep them in my professional life and surround myself with happy and fun-loving people in my personal life.

Living a more balanced life involves taking the time to stop, listen, and focus, because all the answers we seek are there, waiting for us to embrace them. When you know your truth, then you have a choice: you can change it, accept it, or let it go. Remember that there is no right or wrong answer, only what's right for you. Successful weight management is all about you being the authentic you 24/7. Making time for the self is the key.

With that said, we know that maintaining a healthy body is best for our overall health, so why don't we follow through? What's stopping us from doing that which we know is best for us? It's simply that we overcompensate for not being where we want to be. Weight management is about expending more energy than we take in, so why do we have difficulty? We must look at the reasons for us turning to food as a coping tool. What are you pushing away? Simply be still and listen, and you will have the answer you seek. Here is Perl's story.

Perl struggled with her weight for many years. She had one child, and her unhealthy relationship with food went away. Her food choices did not change; however, her desire to self-medicate with food stopped. Each time the feeling came over her to have a baby, she said yes instead of pushing it away with excuses such as "I'm still single" or "I can't afford a baby," or "I don't own my own home," or "I don't have a stable job." She simply accepted the fact that she was pregnant and had to have this baby. This was her only child, who is now a grown woman. When I say giving birth, it does not always translate into having a child. In Judy's case it was about her teaching yoga. We all have something to give birth to, and once that's done, we will not have to worry about our weight again because we are now living on purpose. For Perl it was having a child, for Judy it was teaching yoga, and for me it was writing this book. Living on purpose inspires us, and when we are feeling inspired, we eat nutrient-rich foods that nurture our minds, bodies, and spirits. It's about living the life we are here to experience.

With the recognition and acceptance of our true talents and gifts, with accepting that we do belong here, with being comfortable in our own skins, the weight will melt off with little effort on our part.

Fitness

We can't talk about health without addressing fitness level. It's been said that fitness relates to the quality of being able to fulfil a particular task, be it mentally, emotionally, physically, or psychologically. For me, health means free of disease, but its partner fitness relates to one's physical stamina while involved in physical activities. It's about being able to power walk for hours on end without tiring. I believe weight and many health issues can be reversed simply by just being physical, mentally, and emotionally fit.

I have come to understand that if I want to look and feel a certain way, then I must make an effort to make it happen. There are lots of people who can eat whatever they want and still remain lean and healthy. I'm not one of those people. I can either complain about how fat I am, or I can go for a walk or participate in some form of physical activity that increases my heart rate. The choice is entirely mine. I can complain or make a change today. If I don't make a change today, then I will be in this same position day after day, year after year, feeling the same as I do today. It's my choice. Unless someone is holding a weapon to your head, you are responsible for the way you look and feel today.

Bad things happen to good people like us every day. We can let it defeat us, or we can do something about it and turn it into fuel that motivates us. Sometimes we have to say, "Stop. Enough is enough. I'm tired of living this way." The Toronto Blue Jays baseball team, during its championship 1992 and 1993 seasons, had this quote posted above the tunnel leading to the baseball field: "If it's to be, it's up to me." We all have free will to think and act within our best interests. In order to make things happen, we must dig deep within ourselves to find the motivation necessary to make changes for the greater good.

According to John Winterdyk, PhD, and Karen Jensen, ND, authors of *The Complete Athlete*, "Motivation involves a determination to achieve your goals and to follow your passions, and a commitment to be your best." It's extremely important that we regularly remind ourselves of what's important to us and carry on.

Physical exercise is not only beneficial for managing weight and personal health; it's also beneficial to the nervous system and the circulatory system, and it improves hormonal balance and aids in the metabolism of fatty acids. Aerobic exercise conditions our heart and circulatory system. Blood sugar levels will be stabilized, and your brain will function normally. Exercise also improves your body's balance, coordination, and symmetry.

As a case in point, I recently took a week off work because I was feeling exhausted. During this week I ate healthy and got back into my power walking after a long winter season. On the last day of my vacation, I was walking past a store front for rent, and I thought it was a perfect spot for my office. I didn't have a pen, so I used my phone to take a picture of the sign in the window so that I could contact the real estate agent.

When I got home, I pulled up the picture. My reflection was

in the glass, and I was surprised as to how amazing I looked. I looked like I had lost about 10 pounds, which was not reflected on the scale. A few days later one of my regular customers asked me if I had lost weight, and I responded, "I wish." This new look of mine was a result of physical exercise. When you are involved in physical exercises that raises your heart rate for 20 to 30 minutes two or more times per week, then you build up more muscles that burn fat even faster. On top of that, fat is more bulky than muscles, and therefore I appeared to be smaller than I was. Not only did I look good, but I also felt amazing mentally, emotionally, and physically. I felt fresh and alive in mind, body, and spirit.

I'm not a technical person; however, I feel that in order to fully understand the benefits of daily physical exercise, one must get a little technical. Please bear with me—it's only a few pages. Let's start with the basics. What is exercise?

Some forms of exercise emphasize endurance, others help you become stronger, and still others increase your balance and flexibility. Cardiovascular or cardiopulmonary fitness (the strength of your heart and lungs) is critically important to your overall health. Exercise is sometimes categorized as either aerobic or anaerobic. Aerobic exercise refers to activities that increase your heart rate and thus require you to use oxygen continuously over a period of time. This type of exercise strengthens the functioning of the heart, lungs, and blood vessels. Standard aerobic activities include walking, running, cycling, and swimming. Anaerobic activity involves intense, short bursts of effort, including strength or weight straining, sprinting, and callisthenics. These types of exercise build strength through the demand on the muscles more than the heart and lungs.

With regular exercise, there are as many benefits as there

are people on this planet, some of which we touched on earlier. Below are the top six benefits of why we must move our bodies as much as possible. Most people tell me they hate exercise, and to that I say, "It's because you are not having fun." Find a few things you enjoy and have fun doing them, and you will definitely stick with them. Schedule them into your day, and they will soon become habit.

1. The mind-body connection has been around since the age of the Greeks. Hippocrates is reported to have prescribed exercise for patients with mental illness. Aristotle saw happiness as the supreme good, with everything else in people's lives a means to an end. Homer said, "A healthy mind is a healthy body." The pursuit of happiness is closely linked with one's experience of the quality of one's life. Happiness or a sense of well-being is the absence of negative mood, the presence of positive feelings, and high levels of life satisfaction. Exercise has a direct influence on mood, the perception of stress, physical health, and the sense of life satisfaction.

In 1900 almost all people died of acute infections. Today nearly all of us will die from chronic diseases that in large part are the consequence of an unnatural lifestyle. On average, we burn off 800 fewer calories per day than our parents did.

During the 20th century, exercise was referred to as a "gateway" revolution. The first health-care revolution intended to wipe out infectious diseases. The morality rate changed dramatically with the various discoveries and changes in practice around sanitation, immunization, and vaccination against pandemic diseases. The second revolution focused on eliminating degenerative diseases, and as a result longevity increased.

The third and current revolution is the focus on health and wellness as compared to disease. In the year 2013 prevention is vital for the survival of the human race. Research has shown that physical and mental health benefit from regular physical activity. As a result, exercise increases well-being and contentment. Learn from past challenges and then let them go; have hope and optimism for the future, as well as a steady flow of happiness in the present. Exercise is called a "gateway" behaviour because when you exercise, you feel good, look good, and think well.

2. Exercise is good for your head as well as your heart. It's the magic drug that makes you feel happy when you are sad, settles you down when you are stressed, calms your fears, and increases your self-esteem.

3. Regular exercise energizes your mind and body. There's a physical and psychological change that takes place in exercising people's bodies that goes by the technical term "the feel-good effect."

4. Exercise is mentally effective due to its intimate relationship between physical activity and mental health. As you exercise, you understand your own mind-body connection more completely in relation to:

    A. Brain chemicals—The release of endorphins, the chemical agents within our brains, explain the positive mood that occurs with exercise.

    B. Cognitive, mental, and psychological hypotheses—

People who exercise regularly have higher self-esteem and a greater general sense of accomplishment, as well as an increased sense of self-mastery, self-efficacy, and self-esteem.

C. Combination and interactions—The increased relaxation and sense of comfort in your body may mean that you are less tense, are friendlier, and have natural conversation in your interactions with others.

5. "Exercise and Depression," a study that statistically summarized 80 studies of exercise and depression (North, McCullagh, and Tan 1990), reached the following conclusion: Exercise was a beneficial antidepressant both immediately and over the long term. Regardless of gender, exercise was equally effective as an antidepressant. These conclusions suggest that exercise has both short-term and long-term effects, and it's helpful in reliving depression. The more unhealthy you are, the more of a positive impact it may have, and if you are depressed, a combination of exercise plus coaching or counselling is most helpful.

6. Exercise helps self-esteem. Self-esteem relates to our capacity to function with adaptability within society and to feel in control of our lives. So how does exercise fit into the discussion about self-esteem? What's the connection between exercise and self-esteem? How does our judgment of ourselves relate to our level of physical activity? Exercise makes you feel good, and feeling good then increases your self-esteem; therefore, exercise improves self-esteem.

WEIGHT AND CAREER

Searching for Purpose

How is your chosen career affecting your weight today? Is your job making you fat? The way you feel about the work you do directly affects your weight. When you love, enjoy, and feel passionate about the work you do, you eat nutrient-rich foods that nourish your mind, body, and spirit. When you don't, then you overcompensate by numbing your feelings with unhealthy eating habits.

Living on purpose inspires us, meaning that when we are doing the work we are born to do, then we are able to maintain our weight with great ease because we are eating to live and not living to suppress our lack of focus and direction in a chosen career.

There are millions of books on the market today on career planning, and this is not one of them. My intention here is to get you focusing on your life's work. Identify that special gift that you have for being of service to others, which as a result feeds you soul and results in authentic love, joy, and happiness that can only come from within.

While working as a weight management coach, I came to

understand the connection to our career choices and our weight. I've learned that our unhappiness with the size and shape of our bodies is the direct result of our career choices. When we are in a career that we truly value, then we are happy with how our physical bodies look and feel. In doing what we love feel, passionate about, and have fun doing, we experience a natural high that reduces our appetite for food.

Career is more than just making money to pay the bills; it's really about our soul's desire to be of service to others. I know what you are thinking: *What does that mean?* As humans we are all born with a specific set of challenges to be experienced, learned from, grown, mastered, and developed into a blueprint for helping others heal in mind, body, and spirit. I believe that the moment we tap into this wealth of knowledge, we will find the key to our weight issues, resulting in successful weight management.

Life is about knowing who you are and where you belong. Who you are? Where do you want to be? What's your gift to the world? What must you do to achieve this? You experience certain challenges to uncover these facts. The fact that you are experiencing pain tells you this is not your soul's desire; it's not where you belong. We needed to experience these issues to grow as people. Another way to look at pain is as a GPS system constantly directing us in the right direction.

Based on my research with hundreds of women over the past seven years, I've found that we are overweight due to our attempt to self-medicate. Suppressing the pain of not living on purpose is one reason some of us overeat. In some cases we are confused on what direction to take. Others have major issues with funding the dream, resulting in excessive weight gain. It all comes down to a deep-rooted need in our souls to be of service.

In this chapter we will examine the elements of career satisfaction, including the following questions: What's the truth behind my weight gain? Who am I? Where do I want to be? What's my gift to the world? What must I do to achieve success? What tools do I need—be it education, finances, clarity, desire, or commitment—to get the job done?

Life Lessons

There are two parts to the effects our career have on our weight. The first part is "Lacking the knowledge of our true calling and purpose in life." It's when we are struggling to answer the following three questions: Who am I? What do I need? Where do I belong professionally? The second wave occurs when we do have the knowledge, skill, and experience for carrying out our life's purpose but are not living it. That's when we set out to answer the following question: What's preventing me from living on purpose?

Let me start off by saying our lives are an incredible journey to be enjoyed in the present and to its fullest. When we are present in the here and now, we are then blessed with incredible knowledge from people, places, and events that arise each day, reminding us of what we must do to achieve peace, harmony, and lasting happiness within the self. As mentioned earlier, I've moved several times from country to country and from town to town. One thing I've learned is that all that moving did not make me any happier; in fact, it left me even more confused as to who I am, what my goals are, and where I belong. In the end I realized that everything I've ever wanted is right in front of me.

In finding self, the only way is to travel within for the answer. No matter where in this big, beautiful world you go, the answer you seek is in the same place: *within you.* The question then is, are you really ready to face the truth of who you really are, what your life purpose is, and where you truly belong?

It's okay when we find ourselves in the position of questioning our roles in life. Through talking and listening to others, we will find that we are not alone. We might be at different points on this journey, but we can still learn from each other's experiences and points of view. We are where we are, going through these challenges, so that we can learn and grow as individuals. It does not matter how wide and far we travel; we still have to do the work within. When we learn these lessons, the pain we were experiencing disappears. In other words, when we truly accept who we are—our purpose and where we belong—the excess body fat will fall off without much effort.

As humans we tend to stress ourselves when things don't go our way. Well, there is no need to overplan our lives; we simply need to know what we truly want out of life, set the intention, and then relax; it will come to us at the appointed time. Dr. Wayne Dyer, author of *How to Get What You Really, Really, Really, Really Want,* says that "in order to get what you want you must first wish for it, then ask for it, then set the intention to create it, and finally approach it with passion."

It's my belief that things that are meant to be will be, so there is no sense worrying. It's not about what you want right now, but what you need in order to serve the universe and feed your soul at this time. It's not about planning your life—it's about *living* it.

This got me thinking about all the worrying I have done over the past year. I have made a lot of what I call sound decisions over the year, most of which have not worked out. So what? I did the best that I could in that moment. Worrying and beating myself up with food won't help; in fact, it will only hurt me even more. Worrying also prevents me from being in the moment, resulting in missed opportunities for people coming into my life. Some of my decisions did not work out because it's not the right time, place, or situation for me at that particular time. Sometimes one has to roll with the punches, walk through open doors, and leave locked ones alone. I've learned that when I'm patient, I soon see why it did not work out. In looking at my decision to go on yet another diet, I realize that it's not about losing weight; it's about living on purpose. Putting on weight simply reminds me to focus on my path. I usually put on weight when I am resisting my truth. When I'm working too much to make money to pay the bills, I lose focus of my true destiny. I'm simply putting too much of my energy in the wrong direction. Yes, I do need to make a living, but I don't have to kill myself for money. I need to spend less time worrying about things that do not matter, and spend more time focusing on studying, writing, and teaching weight management for the purpose of living a strong, lean, healthy, and balanced life.

I used to think that all I wanted was to have control over my own life and destiny, which I believed would bring me peace, happiness, and serenity. I no longer feel that way; experience has taught me that when I try to control a certain part of my life, I simply push it even further away, causing more hurt, disappointment, and pain. And as a result I would turn to food for comfort, resulting in an obese body and thus keeping me away from my true calling. This kind of thinking caused me to feel like a gerbil on a wheel in her cage, spinning around and around and not getting anywhere in life. I understand that this is a perfect universe, with everything happening according to divine timing, yet I was still searching for a sign that everything was going to be all right instead of looking further within myself. I now know that it does not matter where my travels take me, how many self-help books I read, or how many psychics I see. I won't find the answers until I stop self-medicating with food and look within; then and only then will I find true joy, happiness, and fulfilment.

Your thoughts will determine whether or not you are going to be happy. If your thoughts are constantly on how miserable your life is, then all you will get is an unhappy life filled with disappointment and pain. Sometimes you are not supposed to see what is going on, but rather you should experience it. It's amazing how surrendering to what is can make someone much happier. Try it sometime; it will definitely work.

If you stop obsessing about your future, you will keep grounded in the present, resulting in connecting with synchronicity and your intuition. The more I tried to control areas of my life, the more confusion and pain I experienced, which always resulted in excessive weight gain. The releasing of my obsession over my career dissatisfaction has eliminated the confusion and pain that I have been experiencing over the past several years. If you are patient, then all will be clear at the appointed time, and then you will receive spiritual guidance about what to do next.

Moving to Vancouver is one example of my recognizing and accepting spiritual guidance. It all started on November 6, 2002. After being off sick for four days, I went back to work and found out that Kimberly, the supervisor, would be visiting the store the following day. As usual, Ava, the store manager, was extremely stressed in preparing the store for this visit, and she made everyone around her stressed as well. Ava had suggested that I come in earlier than my scheduled shift. I thought to myself, *Yeah, right.* I was not about to come in any earlier than I had to for two reasons. First, I hated my job due to a lack of job satisfaction. Second, I was not fond of Kimberly because

I felt she had ignored me during my first five months with the company. By her actions, she told me that now that she had hired, me there was no reason for contact.

That night I went to bed at 1:00 a.m. as usual. I awoke at 5:00 a.m. having what I called a panic attack, which I had not experienced before. I lay back in bed on my back and started the deep-breathing exercises that I'd learned five years ago in a beginner's yoga class. This caused me to fall back asleep. I woke up an hour later and said, "I am moving to Vancouver. It's time." I felt extremely excited and fulfiled after uttering those words; I could hardly contain myself.

I had not been to that province before. My thoughts on the province were, *When I retire, I will move there because of the great weather all year 'round.* Then I recalled approximately five years ago, while at work, I met a lady from Vancouver. During our conversation I'd mentioned my love for hiking, and she'd told me that Vancouver was the best place to do that. I'd decided that for my next vacation in the spring I would go there, but I did not follow through with those plans because I'd lost my job and decided to go back to school full-time. That decision left me with little income to take a hiking vacation.

My new excitement was so great that I went into work early and told Ava that I had decided to move to Vancouver. She was surprised and asked if I know anyone there. I said no, but I felt that it was where I needed to be right now.

After several interviews with my regional manager, Vancouver's regional manager, and the director of sales, my transfer with the company was finally granted two days before I left. It did not make any difference whether or not I got the transfer—I was definitely going; in fact, I had actually found an apartment. I went back to Toronto, packed, and moved one week later.

For some of us, moving is like a drug. When things get a little tough, instead of staying and fighting, we pack up and move on to the next place. This always makes us feel better, but unfortunately in most cases it's short-lived. The next time you are thinking of moving, ask yourself why. Why are you leaving where you are? Why are you going to the next place? Have you learned the lesson you are here to learn? How will your life be different with this move?

I have learned to welcome my challenges, because if everything happened the way I planned, then I would not have uncovered and reached the authentic Althea. It's like peeling an onion: you have to peel off the dead layers, cry to release the emotions that are stuck, and then enjoy the beautiful taste underneath.

It's best to allow things to die naturally. What's the rush? Avoiding attachment to what you think things should be like will result in fewer disappointments. Go after what you are passionate about and don't worry about things that are out of control; it's all about divine timing, so be patient, and you will know what to do next when the time is right. It's not just waiting for the universe to show you the sign—it's also about learning the lessons so that you can move on to the next event in your life when the time is right.

Challenges help to make you stronger and build character. Think back to a point when you were having a difficult time in your life, and then think about how much better your life was when the problem was solved. Don't be afraid to look to the past for comfort; just don't dwell on what you cannot change. Being ashamed of the past is rejecting your today. Yesterday made you the person you are today. You cannot enjoy the future if you don't know where you have been and how you got to where you are today.

The key to finding out who you are, your purpose, and where you belong is to let go and forgive yourself and others for any hurt and disappointment caused. Forgiveness is about lightening your burden and moving on. Your excess body weight is a tool telling you to let go of the past and embrace the present. When you forgive, you make room for happiness in your life. Forgiveness is a way to cleanse your heart and soul so that you can start over. Crying is a great way to release suppressed emotions and open up your heart to make space for both giving and receiving love and forgiveness. It's not about forgetting; it's about forgiving the person so that you can find personal happiness.

Replacing that negative energy with positive energy will give you the strength and motivation you need to use your talents to help others. This will also give you the courage to do what makes you happy, including gaining financial independence, buying a new home, and building strong and positive relationships with your soul mate and friends.

By listening to my body and my intuition, and by eating foods that are nourishing to my mind, body, and spirit, I have found more clarity and direction on how to use my life to benefit others. I am more at peace when I am listening to my soul and to the universe without reservation or attachment to the outcome. I could not have achieved these things if I was being held back with anger and hatred. Forgiveness is about release. Forgiveness is for your sake, not the other person. Forgive and release negative behaviours as a great way to manage your weight.

Life has taught me that I was born with all the answers to the questions about my career path. All the solutions to my challenges are all locked inside of me. To uncover the answers, I have to take responsibility for my behaviours. I must own up to my actions and reactions, as well as accept that this is part of my journey as a spiritual being in a human form.

The lesson of patience will allow me to slow down to hear and see guidance, increase my ability to see and hear signs and messages from the universe, and encourage the development of a much stronger intuition. Ultimately patience will give me the peace, happiness, and serenity I seek in my career. I will know peace when I slow down and live in the moment.

When you are patient, you might have said to yourself that since the Bible says, "God will help those who help themselves," and, "Ask and ye shall receive," then why are your prayers not being answered? They *were* answered—you just don't realize it because you were too busy trying to get ahead. The signs could have been in the form of someone who showed up to help you, but you were too busy to see what they were offering. It might have been that it's not the right time for these prayers to be answered, or that you must feel the pain in order to appreciate and celebrate your successes in the future. Or the answer might be for you to keep asking, and it will be answered at the appointed hour. You won't see the signs until you slow down and start living in the moment, so start today. Take a moment each day and smell the roses; see how much brighter and clearer your day will become.

Get excited about your challenges, because without them, where would you be? Who or what would you be? I have found that my challenges are my best and most effective teachers. We are all here on earth for a reason. The challenges that we are going through on a daily basic get us on the right track of finding our true purposes on earth. I look at my past challenges as lessons in preparation for the future; I don't look at them as an ending but rather the beginning of the next phase of my life.

It's a way for me to move on without guilt or fear of leaving a comfortable situation.

All the struggles we have had and are facing today are in preparation for our true destinies. The way we were conceived is not an accident. It doesn't matter if you were conceived out of love or lust; we are all here to better mankind in our own ways. It does not matter if we are a Nobel Prize winner or a homemaker. We are just as important to mankind.

All the challenges that I have been experiencing have the same message, and that's for me to slow down and look around, because everything I seek is right here. It's the universe asking me, "What's the hurry?" It's also a reminder that this is my life, not a race; there is no finish line, and there are no winners or losers. I should sit back and take in life. I was moving through life at a rapid speed because I wanted to be important, which I believed would result in others giving me love, appreciation, and the feeling of being cherished. I was craving the attention I did not receive as a child.

I don't regret the challenges that I have faced in the past or the ones that I am experiencing now, because these are lessons my soul must learn on earth. Each and every day, I remind myself that binging on large amounts of unhealthy foods limits my potential and prevents me from getting to know myself.

One early afternoon while power walking, I came to the realization that one of the main lessons I am here to learn is how to deal with all forms of losses and death. After looking back through my life, I finally realized what my entire life lessons meant. Death and losses are *for a new beginning,* not an ending. This is how the universe communicates to me that I have learned a particular lesson, and it's now time to move on and start something new.

On a personal level, when Papa died, it gave me a chance

to bond with Mama, Uncle Ed, and my cousin Sophia. Mama's death was meant for me to leave Jamaica and get to know my mother and siblings. Mama's job as a surrogate mother was over. With Mom's death, it was for me to start examining my purpose in life so that I could embrace my true gift of helping others.

On a professional level, when Collacutt, the UCS Group, and Just Kids—the companies I worked for—went bankrupt, it was the universe telling me that there were other experiences for me to embrace, so I should open my eyes. When I did, I then saw the Gap, which opened my eyes and put forth the challenges I needed in order for me to explore my interests in coaching, counselling, emotional wellness, spirituality, and proper nutrition. This step then led me to uncover my passion in life through lessons on emotional issues and how to find my purpose. As painful as all these losses were, they led me to where I am today.

How do you see your life challenges? Do you use them as an excuse to binge eat and suppress your gift, or are you using it as a fuel in helping others?

Teachers come in all forms and sizes, and many times they are least expected. On Saturday, May 10, 2003, while on my way to the bank for the store, I was drawn into Chapter's Book Store. I didn't know why I was there, but I went to the self-help section. On a table the book *The Saint, the Surfer and the CEO* by Robin Sharma jumped out at me, so I bought it. After reading the book, I finally realized the wonderful lessons that my family had taught me even before I was born, and I knew that these lessons were special gifts. This is how I interpret his book according to my life.

The special gift I received from Mom (the saint) was seeing someone who was selfless, who gave of herself, and who loved helping others without the expectation of something in return. Mom died around the same time as Lady Diana and Mother Theresa—all three within days of each other. In my option she answered yes to the question, "Did I serve greatly?"

Papa (the surfer) was very loving and spent most of his time showing me love. Did he love well? Yes, with great commitment and passion. He was a quiet man of great intelligence. He did not feel the need to show how smart he was, or proclaim that he was the leader of the family. He was a man who preferred to stay in the background.

Mama (the CEO) took the time to talk to people. She was a leader in the community during August morning celebration (Jamaica's independence day). She was well-liked and respected. Did she serve greatly? Yes, and she enjoyed every minute of it. She was always the life of the party. I got my high tolerance for alcohol from her!

If I knew what I did about my path here on earth and the lessons learned along the way, then why did I still feel stuck? Why couldn't I figure out what to do with my life? Well, I was not moving forward in life because I was standing in my own way with destructive thoughts. I could not see my purpose because I'd convinced myself that the narrow concept of nutrition and emotional wellness, and nothing else, was what I was here to do. I was trying to push my own agenda out of fear, instead of listening to the universe, my heart, and God. If I would just listen without interruption, then I would see that nutrition and emotional wellness are only one part of my purpose. With patience, when the time is right, I will know the next step. I will then know exactly what action to take to accomplish this. I will know what steps to take when I stop pushing ahead and start paying attention to my guides and intuition.

Through learning certain lessons, we meet certain people

in a particular place and at a specific time. These people's roles are simple: to show us how far we have come and how much work is still needed. I received confirmation of this one evening when I was at home and bored. I turned off the television, went to the mall, and bought a watermelon from the fruit store. I also intended to return a purse that I'd purchased last Saturday. At the last minute I put the purse down and decided not to return it.

On my way to the mall, I felt very hungry, so I asked the angels to please only allow me to eat foods that would nourish me. I then decided to go to Chapters because a few minutes earlier I'd picked up a letter in the mailbox stating if I renewed my rewards card, I would save five dollars.

When I arrived at Chapters, the book *Healing Dreams* by Marc Ian Barbasch was on the clearance table, and it caught my attention, so I picked it up. I then went to the self-help section. Another book on dreams caught my attention, so I put down the one in my hand so that I could pick it up. I then accidentally knocked onto the floor *Come on, Get Happy* by Jonathon Lazear. I picked it up to put it back on the shelf, but it fell out of my hand and onto the floor again. I took it as a sign that I must buy it, so I did. I then went to look at the health magazines. After browsing, I picked up two that were all about spas. After flipping through them, I thought to myself, *Working as a counsellor at a resort would be great, but that's not what I am to do with my life.*

At the register I asked the cashier the cost of renewing the card, and she said, "It's $15 if you are a teacher, and $20 if you are regular. Are you a teacher?"

I said, "Not yet, but I am sure it's in the cards for me in the future." I then saw myself teaching. Emotional wellness through nutrition is definitely what I was to teach the world. I knew what

I was to do—the next step was to receive confirmation as to how to accomplish this without attachment to the outcome.

There is a theme here, in that I am constantly trying to convince myself that I found my way in life, and that I have found my true calling and then do nothing about it. I do nothing about it because I have not figured out how to get there, so I constantly think about how unhappy I am. I am living too much in the future instead of the present moment. I was consistently looking forward instead of experiencing the here and now. I look at the future as a way of using unhealthy foods to ignore or escape from my pain—the pain of being lonely, fearful, and unloved.

I sometimes use boredom as a way to escape and as an excuse for not following my path and life's purpose. Boredom is fear of moving forward; it's when you are doing something that you have absolutely no interest in at that particular time. You are doing something that is non-stimulating to avoid making a change to move in the right direction. This was a way to avoid my true nature and direction, to not listen to the universe, to not live on purpose or serve mankind. Boredom is also a sign that I am not being productive with my time. I am not doing enough with what I know. It's one thing to know, but it's another thing to take action on want I know. I need to pay close attention to what is happening inside and outside of me at that moment, because the answer that I have been waiting for is here; I simply need to open my eyes and hands to receive without judgment.

Thinking can only take me so far. It's now time to put into action what I know, because success comes from taking action. If I want career satisfaction, then I must do what I love by implementing Healthea Solutions to help women manage their weight, improve their health, and develop through coaching.

Counselling is a happy side effect. Boredom is a metaphor to get up and move, to create movement within.

As a result of being impatient, I have a problem listening to the universe for guidance and in taking advice from others who in turn don't listen to me, which makes me angry and withdrawn. Why talk if no one cares or is willing to listen to me? If I am not listening to my own internal dialogue, then why should anyone listen to my external dialogue? The best way to deal with this is by listening to my own inner thoughts, wisdom, and feelings. Then I ask myself, "What am I not paying attention to in my life?"

On a consistent basis I have very vivid and detailed dreams. I now pay closer attention, carrying out the instructions regardless of how I feel about following these teachings. It's my belief that my dreams are divine guidance and will become clearer each time I follow them. I have been searching for guidance outside of me, but most of the answers are coming to me through my dreams. The universe gets my attention by communicating with me through my dreams and music, because music is what feeds my soul by calming me down enough to sense what's going on.

Life Passion

For a very long time I knew I had a special gift to be shared with the rest of the world. What I did not know was exactly what this special gift was. I always felt that this special thing will explain who I am, why I'm here on earth, and to what I belong. I also felt that I got this special gift from Mama before I was 12 years old. This is what I am to pass on to the world; this is what will make women happy as they celebrate life.

The answer was found in these questions: Who are you?

What are you? Where did you come from, and why? How do you look and move forward? This is why Mama had to raise me. After Mama died, a friend of hers told me, "Now that Miss Rose is gone, you have to carry on for her." I did not understand at the time, but now I do. Life is about letting go of your limiting beliefs and fears and embracing your true gifts. Surrender to the power of the universe and watch your power bloom like a flower. Life is all about letting go of your limitation beliefs, thus embracing your true gifts.

I have been working on myself very hard, and on May 9, 2003, it all became very clear to me. I was trying to understand who I was and what my purpose was. *How may I serve the universe?* During this process I learned that the feelings of being stuck and being stifled that I had been feeling for the past 11 years were unresolved issues from my childhood. I was mourning the loss of my childhood by rebelling against my responsibilities, as well as by avoiding my true calling in life.

I had a lot of great ideas of what direction I wanted to take, but I lacked the drive and passion to carry through with these ideas. This was where the rebellion came in. As a child I lost Papa when I was 5 years old; he was the only person I could remember giving me unlimited affection and his time. All the other authority figures in my life loved me but did not tell me verbally. So here I am at 39 years old, not knowing how to show my affections for others and not being able to nurture myself.

This lack of self-nurturing is evident in my weight gain each time there is a major change in my life. I viewed these changes as something like Papa dying and abandoning me all over again. I realized that when my safety and security is threatened, I go looking for food. It's like my security blanked.

In my desire to have a clearer understanding of my life and my role in it, I realized that I must *nurture* myself instead of waiting for someone to do it for me. Papa did his job, and it's now time for me to take over this role by taking responsibility for my own actions today.

To nurture means I must provide myself with sustenance to strengthen my physical body, to train and educate myself in order to grow spiritually and emotionally, and to develop and cultivate myself. I must complement myself for a job well done, such as a pat on the back and saying, "Way to go, great job."

Being more receptive to new ideas in self-discovery and spiritual changes without fear will lead to happiness. When you are nourished. you will be able to become free. You must speak your truth and the need for eating to cover up and suppress your true nature will disappear. You can find more security within yourself when speaking from a place of truth.

While trying to uncover my purpose in life I realized that I was standing in my own way of success by rebelling against my family, because at a very early age I had to act like a grown-up. At 12 years old I was expected to help take care of my four younger siblings. Instead of doing childlike things, I was going grocery shopping with Dad, cooking, cleaning, and braiding my sister's hair. The resentment for being told I had to complete these tasks ran deeply.

In a way I felt robbed of my childhood; I felt rejected and unloved, with a lack of direction in my own life. I was unsure of myself and had low self-esteem. At the time I believed that the separation from my mother at three months old robbed me of my childhood, which left me feeling disconnected from everyone and everything, leaving me unsure of how to go after what I wanted out of life. I was afraid of losing something or someone I loved.

Journeying inward was the only way to uncover the authentic me, my true talents with the blueprint of my life that is predetermined by my soul and God Almighty. Digging deep within has shown me how to deal with my pain, and I learned to forgive family members. I forgave Mom for giving me to Mama and Papa, and for not being there for me when I needed her. I forgave Papa and Mama for taking me away from Mom and then dying when I was 5 and 12 years old, respectively. I forgave Uncle Ken for verbally and physically abusing me. I forgave my stepfather for not being the dad I thought I wanted.

It's really funny—I just realized that the reason I had issues with the above list of people is due to my unrealistic view of them. They did not conform to my idea of who I wanted them to be, and therefore I condemned the person instead of the action. I now acknowledge that they are souls that are on earth to have human experiences, just like me.

When someone acts in a way that is inappropriate to me, then I must ask myself what lesson this person is here to teach me. Facing these past hurts cleared the way for me to move on with my life's work. Going into the past is all about knowing who you are as a person. Knowing how you dealt with situations in the past will help you cope with the issues of today. "Those who don't know their history are bound to repeat it."

With this greater understanding of why I react to others the way I do, I now accept myself exactly the way I am. After all, I am the road less travelled. I am here on earth to experience these challenges. I could have taken the paved road that is very smooth and beautiful on the surface, but I chose the dirt road that is still as beautiful underneath as the paved one. It simply takes some time to see its beauty.

The best way to travel down that road is to look within yourself, at who is to walk your own path, living your own dream, walking to the beat of your own music, and doing what makes you happy. I believe it's up to each person to feed her soul, speak and live her truth, and give and receive love; this is part of living with purpose. This is how you add value to your life and others around you, because you are doing what you love in your own way and at your own pace.

Owning my past has led me to the present and has revealed my purpose in life. I am now able to see that life is full of love because I opened my heart to feel it. I am able to have wonderful people in my life by opening my eyes and seeing them as they are without judgment. I have received guidance each time I opened my ears to hearing them without fear. I experienced beautiful smells by simply standing still to smell them and allowing truth to be spoken. I will no longer run away from nurturing others and myself, because nurturing is what I do best through coaching, counselling, writing, and speaking my truth on weight management for a balanced life.

Another method I use in finding my purpose is by asking myself what I need to be emotionally full. This is a great question because as mentioned before, I use food as a way to medicate myself due to my fear of facing my past emotional issues. It's all about examining the past without judgment in order to retrieve answers to the lessons from the challenges, and then using the answers from the lessons to live in the present moment.

Being in the moment is a source of warmth and strength, where you can stay strong and continue to knock on as many doors as possible. Someone will eventually open his or her door and say, "How may I help you?" With this knowledge, you must choose to ignite the fire within you. You must choose to awaken the power within you. It's about bringing your consciousness into being to fulfil your life's work.

All this hard work showed me that what brings a smile to my face is playing shrink. My experiences have taught me to have empathy for people and situations without attaching myself to the situations or people; that makes it much easier to coach and counsel others. I am successful at it by being me; nothing else is needed. This knowledge is a result of my understanding that true freedom is when I am using my authentic voice. If I don't have a voice, then I ask the universe where my voice is. How did I lose my voice? How can I regain my voice? I believe that the reason I felt stuck in life was a result of me losing my voice years ago. I have learned that my voice is a big part of my identity. I speak from my heart with my real voice, with conviction and passion. I am now paying closer attention to myself when I am angry or upset, because I always speak with my authentic voice when I am upset or excited about something. This is when the real voice of Althea appears to speak her truth. These emotions prevent me from editing and questioning the guidance that I am receiving at that moment. Now that I know what this voice looks, sounds, and feels like, I can use it all the time, which will make me feel more safe and secure, thus eliminating the need to eat when not hungry. Regardless of how harsh it might be, the truth must always be spoken because it's exactly the way that person must hear, receive, and react to in learning to own his or her truth.

Finding my voice has taught me that there are no quick fixes for a happy life. The first part of living purposely—which is finding my purpose, my dream, and my destiny—is now completed. The second part is in the carrying out this gift of helping others to find true happiness, joy and fulfilment in managing their own weight.

It's now apparent that my weight issues are a direct result of my feeling lonely and abandoned, and my need for constant recognition, validation, and acceptance from the outside. Instead of looking within, I chose to self-medicate by eating unhealthy, processed foods to avoid doing what I know needs to be done. As mentioned earlier, the only place I will find the answers is within. The best and most lasting motivation comes from within to alleviate the feeling of being stuck and enslaved, unable to move forward and do what I really, truly want in a career that is fulfiling.

Finally, I must find a way to show my clients how to connect their minds, bodies, and spirits. I must show them what they look like from the inside out. Going through the questions listed below will provide insights into the missing piece of their life purposes.

- What is your purpose? Keep in mind that if you can think it, see it, and dream it, then it's real. The hardest thing for most people to do, including me, is figuring out their purpose in life.
- Why are you here on earth? You know that there is something more meaningful that you must do with your life, but what is it?

I believe that answering these questions will help you to find your path, like I did. Through answering the above questions, I learned that I love to attend seminars on weight management and spirituality, read books on weight management and spirituality, coach and counsel others on weight management and spirituality, and talk to individuals and groups about weight management and spirituality. I also love to writing by putting my thoughts down on paper, travelling, walking outside in nature, working at my own pace without interruptions from others, watching TV, and sipping a cup of tea. These are the things that make me the happiest. I know that all is well with the world when I am engaged in these activities.

Happiness is feeling excited about getting up in the

morning; looking forward to the day; being one in mind, body, and spirit; and turning up the music as you are walking. It's feeling a sense of self-worth and a sense of accomplishment, and it's being passionate about something. In my case, it's being passionate about helping women manage their weight for a full and balanced life. Happiness is a state of mind that I enjoy through the opening of my heart. This is how I feel when I am doing something I enjoy.

I have always been passionate about education. As a child I enjoyed going to school because I found all subjects interesting, with the exception of physical exercise. I hated going out for recess; it seemed that it was all a waste of time, and I wanted to get back to learning. I loved school so much that I wanted to be a teacher. I wanted that because it seemed like teachers were authority figures and were respected in the community in Jamaica.

When I arrived here in Canada, I still enjoyed the learning process, except I changed my mind about being a teacher when I was in grade 8 because children in this country did not respect teachers like kids did in Jamaica. There was no prestige in it, no recognition. I now realize that is the wrong reason to go into teaching. I want to teach because I want to help.

I then realized that my greatest asset is the ability to analyze and see things clearly. So why do I continually seek the aid of psychics and self-help books? Well, it's because I have been searching for recognition outside of myself, and what I have discovered is that I must recognize myself first before anyone else can recognize me. Recognition means to validate through the appreciation and acceptance of the self. It's about appreciating who I am, how far I have come, and what I have accomplished thus far in life. It's accepting gifts from the universe. Accept that you are different in a special way. Accept that you are here to make a difference in people's lives. Accept that you can change the world by changing yourself. Accept that you have the answers. Accept that you are angry with others because they are showing you what you dislike most about yourself; it's about you recognizing yourself within them. They are telling you what your soul needs.

I was searching for recognition to validate me, and I searched for appreciation, acceptance, and attention from others; this is the validation I did not get from Mom. It's all about Mom's love. I know that she loved me, but I didn't feel her love. This brought me to the conclusion that it's part of my destiny to help others find the love within them. When we love and accept ourselves for what we are and what we do, then there is no reason to self-medicate.

As an adult, if love is missing from our lives, it's not up to our parents, spouses, or friends to find it—it's our responsibility. Our parents did the best they could with what they knew when we were children; we can't change the past. The only thing we can do is acknowledge how we felt, learn from it, and move on. Today, I am a teacher in a different way. I teach through my writing, coaching, and counselling women on weight management.

Through this process I also realized that I was not living the life I wanted; instead, I was living for others. In the past I became a retail store manager and bought a condo in order to make my mom and family feel proud of me; this resulted in my being depressed for many years. Depression was a sign that I was not following my path, I was not using my talents, I was not doing enough with what I knew, and I was not being productive with my time. This fact made me feel stuck and confused about who I was and what my purpose was. Through all this I learned that I am the master of my own destiny. I alone can and must make the changes necessary for enlightenment.

To know your truth, look into your own eyes. The eyes are the seats of the soul; nothing is lost in the mind's eye. You can't run away from or lose your passion once you own it. My experience led to the transformation of my credibility. In other words, self-belief results in actualization and transformation.

After finding my purpose, I was still lost—what was missing was how to make it a reality. One morning while working out, I asked the universe why I could manifest things like getting sick because I needed a day off from work, or an iced macchiato, without putting any effort into what I was doing. Then it hit me like a ton of bricks: I manifested these things because I was passionate about them. Passion was what I must put into whatever I manifested. You might ask, "What does passion mean for me?" Well, passion is a knowing. You are convinced that it's the right thing at that moment, no matter what anyone else says. You cannot be persuaded. You know you are living on purpose when you don't compromise your integrity and feel great about it. Passion is saying no to everything that contradicts your goals without having regrets or feeling guilty.

As spiritual beings on earth who are meant to experience human emotions, we are consistently being guided along our paths. When we feel confused and stuck, and we are unsure of our paths, it's because we choose to ignore guidance. We might be waiting for someone to come and take care of us or to nurture us. By paying attention to what's going on around us without passing judgment or being fearful, we will be tuned into the universe and the answers to all our questions. All the answers are inside of us, so we should tune into all our senses without reservations. Below are several events that have happened to guide me along my path.

On September 8, 2003, I got a call at home from a staff member, Angela, reminding me that she needed the letter that we'd talked about for our trend event on Sunday. I told her I would bring it over as soon as possible. I then edited the letter on my computer and printed out six copies. I decided to print another four copies for a total of 10.

As I was leaving, I went through the kitchen, and a voice in my head said, "Althea, take the garbage out." I obeyed the voice and took the garbage with me. When I got on the elevator, an Asian man said hello, and I responded with the same. He then asked me if I was going to the basement, I said yes, and he pressed the button for me. I then noticed two Asian women, mother and daughter, and I looked at them and smiled. When the elevator reached the ground floor, the gentleman got off, and I told him to have a good day; he responded the same.

When the elevator got to the basement where the garbage bins were, I got off and told the women to have a great day. After coming back from the garbage bin, I saw the daughter, and she said hello; I responded the same.

When I got to the door leading to back to the building, I saw the mother standing there, and when she saw me she moved in front of me like she wanted to say something. I stopped, and she told me that she had been living in the building for eight years with her son and daughter. She then asked me how long I had been there, and I said it was eight months. She went on to say she might be going back to her country, Taiwan, next year. I told her about hiring an employee who was from there and who had not seen her dad in four years; she missed him terribly. I then told her to have a great day and left.

This might seem like a regular thing that happens in any metropolitan city. Yes, it does happen all the time. With me, the difference is this time the people are Asians. Usually they just ignore me when I say hello, so I stopped saying it. I then realized that these people were here to give me a message from the universe.

Doreen Virtue, PhD, the author of *Healing with the Angels,* states that the number 88 means that a phase of your life is about to end and a new chapter will begin. It's after this event that my purpose came into full focus, with my writing taking centre stage in my life. There is absolutely no doubt in my mind that my path is to be the very best weight management coach I can be. I have a different way of looking at weight than others people in the industry.

There were several other realizations that came into focus. On September 19, 2003, when I was getting ready for work, I started to experience this very strong heart vibration, a feeling of heightened excitement. I had experienced this feeling several times in the past, including when I'd made the decision to move to Vancouver.

The wonderful news about this occurrence was that I could finally put a name to this feeling as well as explain it to others. I now knew that when I was experiencing this very strong heart vibration, it was a warning that something exciting would be happening to me, or that I would make a decision or receive guidance that would dramatically change my life. This usually happened after I experienced a few days of illness; being sick seemed to open up the channel for me to receive messages more willingly, without fear attached to the situation.

It's one of the most incredible experiences when you finally figure out what you really and truly want to do with your life. To say you are happy is the biggest understatement of your life. Knowing who you are and what your purpose is will bring peace, happiness, and liberation.

With my journey within, I discovered that I am passionate

about healing the soul and the spirit, which will in turn heal the body. I healed my soul and spirit by listening to my own inner voice, praying, meditating, and walking to the beat of my own drum. I am on a mission to help women heal their souls and spirits through writing, coaching, and the sheer joy of helping others. This is my passion because this is the root of my happiness. When you know who you are, what your life's purpose is, where you belong, and what your soul needs to be fulfiled, and when you go after it, then you will find true happiness.

My passion is in guiding and supporting others to help themselves and release old emotions. I show them how to rediscover their authentic selves and regain their voices. I am an intuitive healer of the soul and spirit, and It's my intention to find others who need healing.

The soul is the heavenly student, whereas the spirit is the life force that moves you as the teacher. The soul studies and the spirit teaches. I am passionate about sharing my ideas and thoughts of life with others. I serve the universe by inspiring women with my ideas and thoughts; they in turn will inspire me with their own ideas and thoughts.

My path is to walk down the road less travelled, picking up and fixing what's broken. I don't need to know all the details; I have faith and walk straight down the road. Faith is following the yellow brick road so that I can allow this little light of mine to shine brightly. This is how I am to serve the universe, my lord, and more important myself. Having faith in the universe, my angels, and myself is a guarantee that all will be well at the appointed time.

Take a few minutes in a quiet place and close your eyes. Slowly breathe in through your nostrils and breathe out through your mouth. Before moving on to the next chapter, take note of how you are feeling; write down who you believe you are. What's your life purpose? Where do you belong professionally?

Elements of Career Satisfaction

A major part of managing your weight is feeling content and fulfiled within your career. Let's start by pondering your true feels about your career. How do you feel before, during, and after each day at work? Do you feel happy or sad, exhilarated or frustrated? Is this what you see yourself doing for the next 5, 10, and 25 years, and beyond? If not, what do you see yourself doing? Would you say the work you are currently doing is a job or your chosen career? According to *Webster's Dictionary,* a job is a task or activity performed regularly for payment; the dictionary views a career as a chosen profession or occupation. Our career is what we love, feel passionate about, and have fun doing regardless of how much it pays.

With that said, are you working for profit, or for the pleasure of helping someone else in need? It really does not matter if you are a doctor or a dog walker, as long as it brings you joy; it's all about being of service to others. Everyone needs a doctor at some point, and dogs need to be walked every day. We are all born with that special gift of how to be of service, and all we have to do is look within ourselves to see it.

Career satisfaction begins with the knowing and understanding of your deepest desire. It's knowing where you want to be, what you want to be doing, and with whom. It's why you exist in this world. This very moment is the perfect time to figure out what you want to do and what you need to do to get there, by answering a few questions: What makes you happy? What lessons are you to learn before achieving your goal? What message are you to share with others? What will your legacy be at the end of your life? What is your greatest need and desire for you work life? What's your idea of a loving, joyful, passionate, and fun career?

The elements of career satisfaction include knowing with certainty where you want to be, what you want to do, and who will be the recipient of your service. In knowing where you want to be, you must first acknowledge your gift. So, what's your gift? We all have one; it's that special skill that you are born with and that makes you unique and sets you apart from everyone else.

As children, we knew exactly what our life purpose was. We knew why we were in existence, our reason for walking this earth in this body. We knew exactly why we behaved the way we did. Then, due to our upbringing and conditioning, we start to abandon it; as a result we start to experience pain. The further away from our true gifts and natural talents that we stray, the greater our dissatisfaction with our careers. The further we stray from our true calling, the more pain we experience. The more pain we experience, the more we eat to cover up the unbearable pain.

This gift is what makes us different from all other human beings. It's what we are here to contribute to the world around us. How have you been suppressing your true nature? How have you been denying the truth of who you really are and what you are to accomplish in this lifetime? What are you afraid of? Are you afraid that no one will like you, that you will be rejected or made fun of? Why are you resisting your truth? What are you afraid will happen if you do acknowledge and accept your true nature?

Why must we accept the role we are here to play? What if I told you it's to fulfil our souls' desires, and to learn, grow, and teach? Would it then make it easier for you to accept who you really are? According to a *Forbes* Magazine poll, published May 18, 2012, 44 percent of people in Canada and the United States are unhappy with their jobs, and another 19 percent are somewhat dissatisfied. In my practice, it's even higher. When I ask people, "Why do you stay in this unhappy job?" the answer is always the same: "I have to pay the bills." That is fascinating to me because that's the same excuse I used for years. After working with these individuals, I soon realized that the core of all their unhappiness with the work they do is that it's not where they want to be. As a result, they are always angry, show up late for work, take lot of sick time, and binge on unhealthy foods to suppress their true feelings.

When we are doing what we love, then we go to bed so that we can get a good night's sleep. We awake with ease and with lots of energy. We can't wait to go to work in the morning. We enjoy our coworkers and clients. We stay at the job as long as it takes to get everything done, without complaining.

To achieve career satisfaction, we must ask ourselves, "Who am I, and why am I here?" These are question that humans have been struggling with since the dawn of time. As children, we mimic our parents' actions and take on their belief systems. Then as teens we start to pull away, rebel, and sometimes succumb to peers pressure. This is all part of the maturation process in order to become an independent individual. At some point we then pull away from our peers when we realize their way of thinking and acting does not feel right for us. We start to read materials that make us think. We listen to what our elders are saying. We pay close attention to people who are successful versus people who are not. Then in the end we form our own identity based on all the knowledge we have gathered.

It's not that we did not know who we are at birth—it's that with so many different influences, interferences, and opinions of who others believe we are, we turn our backs on our true nature. We then have to take it all in to determine what feels right for us. It comes easy for some of us, but others need more time. The trick is to stick with it no matter what.

When we do something and it feels bad, then it's not who we are. The fact that we are feeling uneasy about doing or saying something is the soul telling us that it's not us. When we feel good, then we are doing that which is in our best interests. We know we have found our way when we only do what's feels right to us. Listening to our souls will lead us to eating healthy, getting lots of rest, and enjoying physical activities that will aid us in permanent weight management. Our career dissatisfactions are designed to get us back on the right track. Over the years I've been asking myself who I would be without my lifelong struggle with my career. How would my life be different? Would I be living the life I'm living now? If not retail, what would I be doing for a living? Where would I be living? Would I have the life that I have today? And that is why we are experiencing these challenges in this moment. This is the lesson we are here to learn from all the people, places, and conditions that exist in our lives today. They all have specific lessons to teach us. What lesson is that? Career is all about being grateful and thankful for what we do have today. Walk into open doors and leave the closed ones closed. Continually pushing on a locked door will only make the door non-responsive. We must work at being of service to others. Don't rush the process; all will be clear soon.

Challenges are the opportunity for starting something new, for change. I'm a very careful and conscious person. Over the years I have learned I like to take time to think, evaluate, and reflect on each situation before I act. When I don't take the time, I feel overwhelmed by the magnitude of the situation. With all that said, it's not the people, places, or circumstances—it's the fact I don't have the time to do a better job.

I pick a horse and ride it to the finish line, no matter how long it takes or what I have to do to stay on track. If I fall off, I will simply get back on without question. The shortest distance between two points is not always a straight line; sometimes you have to take a detour. Sometimes it's to meet someone who will get you to your destination faster, and sometimes it's simply to take a break. Challenges are a good thing no matter how painful. They are designed to show us the way, make us stronger, and make us grow as a person.

One day I was running to get the SeaBus when I noticed the clock starting over from 15:00. I stopped running when I heard the attendant asking me, "Do you want it?" I responded yes, and then she said, "You can make it. Never give up!" This got me thinking about my career goal of being a full-time weight management coach. That simple statement from the attendant reminded me that I must keep the faith. I'm still in retail to prove that no matter what distractions are thrown my way, I can still keep the focus on what's important, and that's to be of service to women on their weight management journey.

Yes, I do know that I'm heavier than I want to be, and that's okay for now because I must learn the next lesson. I believe this lesson is about focusing on my truth. I must not allow a few extra pounds to stand in the way of my success. Once I accept this fact and do what I love, the weight will fall off. I was being reminded that everything that I have learned over the years is to help others heal in mind, body, and spirit. Only in helping them will I help myself as well.

Now what? It all starts with you willingly taking people's frantic phone calls no matter how inconvenient it is for you in that moment. Never give up on your deepest desires; keep plugging away because success is just around the corner.

Recently I found myself sitting in the middle seat on a flight from Vancouver to Toronto. When I booked my flight, I forgot to book a seat as well. I'm most comfortable at the window so that I can see what's going on outside, despite the altitude. As I sat there getting more and more annoyed at myself for the decision of not reserving my seat, I noticed that everyone who had a window seat had the shade drawn. I thought, *Why on earth would you would pay $25 more for a seat, only to hide in the corner sleeping?*

A huge smile came over me as I recognized the fact that this was a metaphor for my life. I moved from Toronto to Vancouver to pursue my dream of being self-employed. Once again I find myself in my old profession retail and hating it. So what am I hiding from? Could it be I'm hiding away from success? Why the hell am I doing this? Why am I hiding in retail? What am I really afraid of? What's really going on? Several times in the past, I've left the profession only to go back within a year because my venture into self-employment did not work out. So what's missing? Where did I go wrong?

My research with numerous clients over the years has shown me that the secret to us reaching our goal weights and maintaining them for life lies in living on purpose. So why am I not doing what I love to do the most, which is studying, writing, and teaching weight management? One time I left my well-paying job to pursuing this dream … only to fall flat on my face. Sleeping in the corner is the same as hiding away in retail and wasting my talent for helping women heal the source of their unhappiness. I'm wasting my gift as a healer.

What am I missing? I'm sure it's right in front of my face, so why can't I see it? What must I do to really see it? Part of me is saying, "Althea, open your eyes and you will see it. Keep looking and you will see it soon. Just a little patience, and you will soon make Healthea Solutions Weight Management Inc. a success." It's important not to give up on our dreams. So it did not work out the last time, That does not mean it won't happen today or tomorrow. This reminds me of the quote, "If at first you don't succeed, try, try again."

Based on my upbringing, it makes sense that I would take it as rejection and abandonment when things don't happen exactly as I want them to and in the projected amount of time. However, that's not the case; it's simply not the right time or place for achieving this goal.

Have you ever had a brilliant idea of what your true calling is? It's so vivid in your mind that there is absolutely no question that this is how you are to serve mankind. Your first instinct is to put it into action right away—only to have it not work out because it's not the right time. That's because it's only part of the puzzle. You are to live with the thought, idea, belief, and feeling for a while. Don't rush the process; instead use this time to sharpen your skills each and every day.

Dr. Phil McGraw, author of *Self Matters,* says that when he gets an idea, he always lives with it for 15 minutes before acting on it. That's sound advice, if you ask me. Again, there is no need to rush the process. Live with it for as long as it takes. Sometimes taking a few minutes—or a day or a month—to mull things over will lead to greater and more permanent success. We must ensure we have all the facts for this venture before putting it into action.

When it does not come together the way we want it to and in accordance to our time frame, it's normal for some of us get angry and frustrated, and then to turn to food to calm ourselves down. In other words, we decide we want something, and when it doesn't happen quickly enough, we bury our dissatisfaction with food. However, we can break this destructive cycle by being patient with ourselves.

My less-than-successful ventures away from retail management have taught me that I do an excellent job of making goals; however, instead of waiting for the perfect opportunity, I take the first offer that comes my way. I'm constantly putting my goals, my action plans, on the back burner! Sometimes it takes time to put all the pieces together. It's like the old proverb, "The baby must first learn to crawl before walking." In other words, first comes the idea, then you research its pros and cons, then you compile action plan, and then you put it into action. I know it's tempting to move from idea to action; however, you must be more patient, and you will be rewarded with success in the long run. I have been struggling to get out of retail management since 2000, because I have been telling myself that it's not very fulfiling, which is true. So I keep moving in and out of one retail store after the other with the same result. I know that I want to help women in a deeper and more meaningful way. I told myself that it was as a nutritionist, so instead of researching it I jumped right into opening an office. Needless to say it was not very successful. Then I convinced myself that it was as a life coach, and again I left retail to open up an office, with the same result. I ended up in retail management again and hated myself even more. True to form, I turned to food for comfort. If I was patient in taking the time to see the big picture, I would have seen the truth. I would have understood that I need to combine my retail management background with my nutrition knowledge, along with my gift of coaching and counselling through the healing process.

Looking back, I can clearly see that it's not the profession I was unhappy with—it's within me. So, Althea what do you need? What's missing within you? What is that whole crying out for within you?

My previous ventures in self-employment were not successful because I did not have all the pieces put together, leaving me confused as to how I'm to serve the world. These setbacks gave me opportunities to find a way to get my clients on track in weeks instead of years. I've always known what I wanted to do; I am simply lacking the knowledge in how to achieve this level of success as a professional weight management coach. I believe these setbacks were the universe's way of testing me on my commitment to making Healthea Solutions Weight Management Inc. a reality!

The last time I left retail to pursue my coaching dream, it did not work out because the coaching world was not ready for me. A lot of time we do say we are not ready; however, I do believe that sometimes it's the world that needs to catch up to our beliefs and ideas on surviving in this universe. With that said, I stayed with that job, and it was the wrong time to make the moves I did.

I was sharing these experiences with a friend, whose response was, "You know what needs to be done, so why are you waiting around and settling instead of going after what you want and deserve?" That's an excellent question. The answer is quite simple: I've learned that it's not that I'm settling, it's that I must be a little more patient. It's about putting all the pieces of the puzzles together. Her next question was, "How will you know when it's time to take action?" I will know because the door will be wide open; all the money, time, energy, and clients I need will be there.

All the signs were there, and I ignored them. Case in point: I was losing weight without trying as I was researching and writing lesson plans for teaching "Life Skills for a Balanced

Life," which was a clear indication that I was on the right track. However, when I found what I thought was the perfect office space, I had difficulty coordinating my schedule with Jim, the owner of the building, to sign the lease. Despite the fact that he told me the space was mine, I was worried that I would lose it, and instead of being patient I rushed the process. Looking back, I realize that this was a clear indication for me to focus on building my client list instead of rushing into an office right away.

When we make the correct choices, we open another door of joy, peace, and happiness. We are overweight because something is missing—we are not living our best life. We are out of balance and are not fulfiling our hearts' desires. It's like a thread: once you identify the core of your unhappiness, everything else will fall into place. For me, it's the relationship with my career.

I believe living on purpose inspires us, and when we are feeling inspired, we eat nutrient-rich foods that nourish our minds, bodies, and spirits. We become alive because we are doing what we love. As a result we are able to reach and maintain our weight goals. The right people and opportunities flow into our lives at the right time without much effort.

These experiences taught me to only walk through open doors and leave the closed ones closed. Temporarily suspending your pursuit of your goal because of circumstances beyond your control does not mean you've failed; it does not mean that you are giving up on your dream. It simply means that there is something else you must do before this can happen. You will quickly learn that part of the puzzle was missing. Regardless of what's happening in your world, always keep your dream alive and at the forefront of your mind. Be ready, because success is just around the corner.

The meaning of success is interesting to me because everyone has a different idea of what it means. The dictionary definition is "the achievement of something we desired or planned for." Regardless of what it means to you personally, why do we freak out and sabotage ourselves when we reach our goals? How many times have you asked for something and received it, only to ignore it? I believe we normally turn our backs because our needs have changed, it's not what we thought it would be, or we don't care for the package in which it arrived. There are also times when we get what we ask for; however, we do not recognize it. Why?

To get what you really want, you must be very specific and clear before asking for it. When I ask for something and do not receive it, the universe is asking me to stop and decide if this is really what I need or desire. If it's what I want, it will happen soon after. If it's not, then it's time to change course. When I was first getting started in business, the hardest part was getting funding. I had the knowledge, skill, and education skill set; all I needed to get started was investment capital. I turned to all the usual avenues for help, with no luck. I thought of giving up many times, but I decided against it in the end. Yes, this is really what I need and want.

When you believe in your vision, it will happen without much effort. Once you determine what it is that you truly want, then the next step is to make a plan of action, water it with patience, and let it grow. Stop chasing your goals and dreams and let them come to you organically.

As individuals we all have our own ideas of what success is. The question is, what is your idea of success? How do you know when you are successful? To answer these questions, you must first determine what you want and then go after it. Keep climbing the ladder until you are not having fun, and then step back one notch; this is your happy zone, your sweet spot.

It's been said that success is when preparation meets opportunity. For me, I believe success happens when you are ready for it. It's believing in something enough to stick with it no matter how challenging it might be. At times we have to fight our way through worry, doubt, and confusion to bring about the change that will lead us to a successful career. Confusion occurs when we have to make certain decisions about moving forward. You get what you believe to be a brilliant idea. You are so excited that your thoughts are consumed with this idea—and yet you do nothing. Are you afraid, and if so, of what? Ask yourself, "What's the price for changing versus not moving forward?"

You know you must make a change, but how do you know when to move forward in the implementation of your plans, as compared to continuing the planning process? It's about being ready to receive. With that said, you will know when the appropriate door is open. Meditation is also an excellent way to go deep within you to where the answer lies.

Doubt and procrastination is the universe double checking to see if this is really the road you want to travel. Are you really sure this is what you want? This is the time for confirming. Do you really want to do this kind of work day in and day out? Will this type of work feed your soul, bring you joy, and provide a source of comfort in good times and in challenging times? This is the time to locate the source of your worries, and you will have your answers. This is my answer to my food abuse and bringing about unsatisfying careers. In the end, not only will you find peace in your career, but you'll also find it in all areas of your life. There is no sense resisting because the only way to be truly happy is to totally accept and use your gift to help others. Again, the more you use your gift to help others in need, the less your weight will become an issue.

For years I've told myself that in my journey to a successful career in weight management, my first step is to lose weight. I now realize it's not about losing weight—it's what the weight is communicating to me, which is that I must focus my attention on purpose. I'm experiencing this pain in the form of being overweight in order to motivate me in moving forward. I'm feeling ignored in this moment because it's time to channel all my pent-up anger and hurt feelings into building a strong, viable business.

I must give others a reason to pay attention. I should give them a reason to stop and take notice of who I am and what I do. My body is telling me I must hold myself to a much higher standard, and others will take notice. "You are the best in this profession, and they won't know this until you show them." It all starts with the decision to be successful! The first rule of success is to make a decision and then take a course of action. When something doesn't work, ask yourself, "What can I do today to make it better? What piece of the puzzle is still missing?"

As we mature in life, we learn that happiness is a state of mind. We can choose to be happy, or we can choose to be miserable. As I'm writing this today, I have a wonderful life. Is it the life I dreamed of? No, however it's the one I've been given. I can choose to focus on what I don't have, or I can give thanks for what I do have today. By sticking to the plan, I will get there soon.

Does that mean I have to give up on my dreams of being self-employed, being happily married, owning my own home mortgage-free, having one million dollars in the bank, and maintaining a strong, lean, healthy body fewer than 124 pounds? Absolutely not!

So what's the point of having goals and dreams if I can't have them immediately? I have dreams so that I have something to look forward to and something to work toward. I believe in my heart of hearts that they will come through one day. In the meantime, my focus is in doing the best job I can with what life brings my way. I'm looking at these challenges and situations as preparation for what's to come. They are preparing me for greatness. Remember, life lessons are designed to teach us who we are and to bring us closer to ourselves so that we can know our true and authentic self. When faced with a challenge, I continue to ask, "What lesson am I to learn from this situation?"

The consistency and persistence of vision is in my commitment and dedication to a successful career in weight management. I have come to understand that having tunnel vision in this area of my life is the only way to get things done: decide what I want, make a plan, and stick to it no matter what else comes up. Even in the uncomfortable moments, I should stick with it because a breakthrough is just around the corner. The author of *The Help* sent her manuscript to 60 publishers before finally getting a book deal, which was then turned into a blockbuster movie.

The biggest career lesson I've learned over the years is simply to stay in one place long enough for my idea seeds to grow. Just what is patience? It's about being in the moment and experiencing what is. It's honouring the presence of others and giving them my full attention. It's about being open and receptive to what is in this very moment. Having goals and dreams are a must, but we must pursue them at our own pace. Rushing the process will only cause pain.

For years I was trying to lose weight, and I did. However,

I was unable to keep it off because of my lack of patience with my career choice. Instead of sticking to my goals, I would get angry, give up, and move on to something else. Needless to say, it always left me feeling even angrier and more frustrated. What I did not realize at the time was that if I was only a little patient and had stuck around, my dreams would come through faster. Passion, dedication, and commitment—that's what I need to be successful! As mentioned earlier, success is preparation and being ready to receive all that which I desire.

My Healthea Solution to life is that everything happens for a reason. Whatever emotion we are experiencing in any given moment—real or imagined, happy or challenging—it is here to teach us a lesson. Look at the people, places, and situations in your life today, and ask yourself, "What is this person, place, or situation here to teach me?" This is how you get to know yourself.

The key is in the knowing that it's not the other person—it's me. They are only mirroring that which I cannot see within myself. They show up in my life in this moment to trigger certain memories and to expose the stories I've been telling myself. My subconscious mind is trying to get my attention, calling me to be present and centreed in my body.

To be truly successful in your career, you must do what brings you fulfilment. That starts with knowing who you are at your core. It's going deep within you and answering the tough questions: What are you good at? What do you love, feel passionate about, and have fun doing? What do you find fascinating? What makes you feel good? In what are you an expert? What can you do today to find opportunities to grow, to meet people, and to be known? Where are you now, and what's next step?

Recognize and accept your true talent and gift. Accept that

you do belong here, it's what you were born to do, and this is where you need to be. When you are comfortable in your own skin, the weight will melt off with little effort on your part.

WEIGHT AND MONEY

The Money-Weight Connection

After years of moving from job to job and company to company, I asked, "Is this all there is in life? You finally got your answer— now what? You have the skills, knowledge, determination, and commitment to follow through on your life's work. So, what's holding you back from making your next move?"

Money. Cold, hard cash. You know you need investment capital to carry out your life's work. Now what? First, you have research how much you need to get started and to keep you afloat for the first year in business. Where can you go for assistance? Who can you turn to for help in getting the financing for this venture? This is where I found myself no long ago. I realized that I did have unresolved issues with receiving and using money in a manner that honoured others. I know it sounds crazy, but it's true.

As you know, money is a very important tool in today's society. We use it in exchange for goods and services, as well as a measurement of our success. I believe most of what we know about money is taught to us by our parents, whether it's directly or indirectly. If they worried about having enough to pay the bills, then chances are we will as well. If they were frugal, then we might be as well. If they were savers, then we might be savers, too. They don't have to talk to you about money for you to pick up their money habits and beliefs. There is always the exception, but for the most part studies have proven this to be fact. These are the goals of this chapter:

1. Understanding your spending habits

2. Discovering where they came from (where, when, and what started it all)

3. Learning how to change these behaviours if you so choose

4. Knowing your spending history

5. Acknowledging your spending habits

6. Stating your intentions for your financial future

7. Planning out how you will get there

Before we get into my money history, let me tell you a little about my family dynamic. I was born in Jamaica and spent the first 12 years of my life there. At 3 months old my mother gave me to her parents to raise. There, I felt very loved and wanted; all my physical, emotional, spiritual, and financial needs were met without me asking for anything. To keep it all straight, I refer to my grandparents and two uncles as my primary family, because I spent the first part of my life with them. My secondary family consists of my mom, stepfather, two brothers, and two sisters.

When I was 5, my grandfather died, and two weeks after I turned 12, my grandmother died. At this time my mother was living in Canada with my stepfather, and she thought it was best that I live with them and my siblings. My earliest memory of how important money is occurred on October 28, 1976, when I arrived in Canada from Jamaica. The day after we arrived in Toronto, my mother asked me if Uncle Ed had given me any money. I then showed her $40 Canadian, which is what I got when I changed my Jamaican dollars into Canadian money at the airport. She asked, "Is that it? You mean that he couldn't sell a cow and give you the money, after all that you did to keep Mama company?" I came to the conclusion that when someone does something for me, they will expect something back in return. It taught me that asking for or accepting help from others has a price to be collected at a later date.

I believe I overspend because of the lack of attention I received from my parents, especially from Mom. Each time I asked Mom for money to buy something, she would say that she did not have the money, which I would internalize as a rejection of who I was. One such example occurred when I asked for a new dress because I was tired of wearing the same two dresses to church, alternating them each week. She said she did not have the money—yet she bought another dress for my sister right after I had asked. Needless to say, it was a very painful situation for me to experience. In her mind she could not show favouritism toward me. In my mind I thought, *Mom loves everyone more than she loves me.* I have to compensate the only way that I know, which is to spend money on myself because I'm the only one I can truly depend on. I was getting $5 allowance each week, which I used to purchase books and food to escape the pain I was feeling. I was trying to cover up and suppress the pain of the rejection I was feeling.

The truth was that Mom loved me more but was afraid to show me, because she feared retaliation from her husband, who often accused her of showing me favouritism. The fact that I was quiet did not help because I did not let her know how unhappy I was; instead I withdrew from her, letting all the anger fester inside me. Each time I ate and spent money on myself, I was showing myself love and acceptance, or so I thought.

After going away to college, I started to notice that I was always running out of money. I was spending more and more of my money on fabric to make my own clothes and buy junk food and books. It wasn't until May 15, 1987, after resigning from the fabric store without lining up another job, that I started to show the after effects of spending more and more money, especially on junk food, which resulted in excessive weight gain and financial instability.

My spending escalated because I was angry and frustrated at the company for its lack of support of the ideas and skills that I had put on the table in order to improve the company. I look at the rejection of my ideas as a rejection of me, just like Mom did. The only way I knew to rebuild my self-esteem was to fill up the hole by spending money on junk food in order to make me feel better for a little while. I felt that I had to buy things for myself to show myself love and to acknowledge my self-worth, because no one else would.

The events that took place at the fabric store brought up three old money memories from my childhood. The first was when Mom told me that Uncle Ed did not give me enough money. The second was when Mom said no to buying me a new dress. The third event occurred the year that everyone in my family received Christmas presents, but I got none. I felt like the forgotten child. During this period of my life, money couldn't get away from me fast enough.

At the same time I also paid off my student loan in full when there was a mix-up with the bank, and they did not get the monthly payment on time. When the bank teller called me at my new job to ask about the payment, and I told her it was there, she then accused me of buying drugs with the money. As someone who has never tried drugs and looks down on those who use, I was insulted. I went down to the bank the next day and immediately withdrew all my savings, paying off the loan so I would not have to deal with her ever again.

Since then, I always spend when I am mad or upset. Buying books makes me feel worthy and acceptable, and food balances my hormones, temporary filling the void and calming me. These spending sprees leave me feeling ashamed and alone when I need the money for something else, such as paying my mortgage and other bills.

My spending patterns have changed over the years. During my teen years, out of all the things that I spent money on, the number-one thing was books. If I was well read and educated, then I would be acceptable. It started out with me reading horror and mystery books to escape my childhood. Today it's self-help books; I search for direction and guidance from the authors. I want them to tell me that I am an okay person, that I am normal, and that there is nothing wrong with me. Am I still trying to escape life? Yes.

I spend money when I am upset; when I am feeling lonely, bored, or confused about what to do next; and when I am searching for guidance. For a brief moment it makes me feel good. I buy stuff that I don't need to collect more stuff, which says I am okay because I have more stuff. I am spending to give myself things that I don't need to show my family that I am successful.

I have come to realize that the more material possessions I accumulate, the more trapped I feel, enslaved to the material world. The only way to get off this money train, whose sole purpose is to collect enough material possession in order to feel worthy of love, is to surrender to the universe so that my true voice can be revealed to me.

In my 20s and 30s my spending pattern switched to food, resulting in a weight gain of 50 pounds on several occasions. Food balances my hormones and calms me. These spending sprees leave me feeling ashamed because I needed the money for something else, such as paying my mortgage and other bills. When and where did I come to the conclusion that spending would make me happy? The more material possessions I accumulated, the more trapped I felt.

In the past the biggest issue was my condo, which I looked upon as a burden and an obligation. The only reason I'd purchased it was to show my family I was successful. What I have done over the years is adopt my secondary family's philosophy of what money is and what it does. It works great for them, but it's detrimental to me physically, mentally, emotionally, and spiritually. This is why I encourage scarcity.

What does money represent to me? Well, it's the freedom to live a life of helping women understand the link between living on purpose and the foods they eat, without worrying about how to support myself financially. It's not about what I want—it's about what I need to be happy and fulfiled in life, which is spending my working hours studying, writing, and teaching weight management to women who are inspired to changing their bodies and ultimately their lives.

Over the past eight months, I have had two separate dreams

about money. The first was of me counting coins so that I could purchase something, which I interpreted as meaning that because I did not have enough money, it was the same as not having all the information necessary to make a decision on my life, whether it's my career, my financial health, my weight, or my relationships. I must be patient because I will meet someone who will show me the missing piece of the puzzle.

The second dream I had said that what I do best is sing. Then when I was awake, I was humming the song "Now That We Found Love." Then I started to daydream about being married and going to a soup kitchen in California with my in-laws as volunteers. I saw an old, black man from Jamaica; I asked him his story and then found him a job. Later we both ended up on Oprah's show, where he thanked me and told me that he started a home for homeless people who wanted to get back on track, and he then won the lottery after this.

What does this dream means? Is it possible that this dream was a heads-up that I would be winning the lottery and that I must use this money to start a home for homeless people who want to get back on track? That might be. Or it's telling me that I must think of what I am doing with my money, and I must be more conscious of where it's going. Money is energy, and knowing where I am sending my money will lead me to my lost, misplaced energy.

That very same day, Wednesday, September 10, 2003, my boss, Carol, bought me lunch, and I was telling her about a call I got from my friend Laurie, who lived in downtown Toronto. She asked me what Laurie did, and I told her that Laurie was independently wealthy. Carol then asked what Laurie did with her money, and I said I didn't know.

That night I was watching the reality show *The Family,* where the man who had control of the family fortune had to make a decision about what to do with the money. He could keep it all for himself or share it with the family. He surprised his entire family (and me) by splitting the money; all 10 members got $100,000 each. Again, the universe was asking me to keep track of my energy and was reminding me that it's better to share what I have with those who are less fortunate.

While I was recording the events of the past 17 hours, the song "A Moment in Time" by Kelly Clarkson came on the radio, and I started to cry because I realized that I was to share my wealth with others. I believe that this is a message from the universe for me to stop holding on to money. By loosening my worry of money, I will attract all the abundance I need in order to live my purpose of helping others without worrying about how to finance this venture. All the monetary gain that the universe is offering to me is to be shared with others so that they can start their own venture for making the world a better place. This ties in with my dreams. My life purpose is not about making money but rather using my abundance to help others. It's about helping women maintain their weight to improve their health and encourage personal development through coaching and counselling, resulting in a fulfiled life.

The most powerful money lesson happened on Monday, July 7, 2003, on my way home from work. I stopped at Ricky's Restaurant for some fish and chips for dinner. While I was waiting, I overheard a conversation between a teenage boy (about 16 or 17 years old) and mall security. The boy had lunch at the restaurant, and when he got the bill, he told the waitress that he'd lost his debit card; she then called security.

When they arrived, he explained the situation to them. He then told them to call his grandmother to come and pay the bill. Security dialled the number he gave them and then handed him the phone. He then told his grandmother that he'd lost his debit card and couldn't pay the bill and that the security guards were going to haul him off to jail. She then told him that she had no way of getting to the restaurant. At this time my order came, and I left without knowing the outcome. On my way out of the restaurant, I chuckled to myself because I thought the boy was trying to scam the restaurant.

When I reached my apartment building and got on the elevator, I thought about the boy at the restaurant and had a good chuckle again. On my way out of the elevator, I dropped my keys, and they fell down the elevator shaft. I called the after-hour emergency number on the office door of the building. The person who answered the phone told me that he would try to get hold of the building manager; if he couldn't, then he would call the elevator company to come and retrieve the keys—for a cost of $300.

I told him I didn't have that kind of money. He promised he would try to get hold of the manager. He called me back an hour and a half later and said that the assistant manager of the other building was on her way to let me into my apartment.

When she met me in the lobby, it was 8:30 p.m. She then told me that I was very lucky because she was usually gone by 4:30.

The next day I called the building manager and told him what had happened with my keys. He said he had to call the elevator people and get back to me. I also asked him to go up and lock my door, because I was now at work. He called back about an hour later and informed me that it would cost me $140 to retrieve the keys. I told him I would pay for it. I then went to the building on my lunch break to pick up the keys and give him a cheque.

That evening when I got home, I decided to pick up my mail. There was an envelope from United Van Lines, the company that had moved my things from Toronto to Vancouver last January. It was a letter of apology for overcharging me, and there was a cheque for $146.86 enclosed. When I told my friend Laurie about the chain of events, she then asked me if I'd had the money to cover the boy's bill at the time, and I said yes. I can't prove it, but I bet that his bill was $6.86. I came to this conclusion because if you add that amount to the $140 it cost to retrieve my keys, that would be the total of the cheque I received from the moving company.

The universe does not punish; it simply teaches lessons in a format that is unique to each individual to ensure the messages are received and understood. This was an opportunity for me to share my money with someone in need. I must look for a way to give money to those who need it. And it's not just about money—it's about my time and energy, which I have in abundance.

It's not about holding on to what you have; rather, it's about releasing trapped energy in order for it to flow consistently. This energy can take many forms, including worrying about that which you know is done and cannot be changed, and being impatient. Financial worries prevented me from having a good time, enjoying life, and moving forward to the next chapter in life. For decades I kept abundance at bay because I was afraid to accept it. Being fearful prevented me from seeing and hearing the truth of who I was and the work I was here to carry out. I used food to drown out my own voice telling me that I must help others heal in mind, body, and spirit.

Abundance is the resource of the universe, and we all have the ability to tap into it. Having abundance in the form of money can be achieved by trusting in our ability to listen and by trusting in the messages from the universe. Then we should follow these messages no matter where they may lead us.

Attracting money is easy when you listen; it is difficult when you don't pay attention to what's going on around you. Be aware of where you are, the people around you, and what's going on. I have found the most effective way for me to be in the moment is by asking myself this question: "How is being here with these people affecting me in mind, body, and spirit?"

I believe it's hard to listen when I'm binge-eating large quantities of junk food. Have you ever asked yourself, "Why am I eating this when I'm not hungry?" I have. Usually my reasoning is to calm myself because I'm receiving some kind of universal message that I don't understand; I'm feeling overstimulated with information. What I now realize is that although it does the trick in calming me down temporarily, it also takes away or stops the messaging process. As a result, I get even angrier and more disgusted with myself for not knowing what to do next, so I go out and spend even more money on things I don't need.

I was reminded how important it is to pay attention to my thoughts in order to understand the message from the universe on Wednesday, October 8, 2003. That day I had an appointment with Gail from Career College at 1:30 p.m. When I woke up, I felt very tired and drained. I forced myself to keep the appointment because I felt that this was something I must do in order to move on. On the sky train, after realizing I was feeling extremely angry, I surrendered my anger to God. When I switched over to the bus, I noticed that I started to feel better.

About 10 minutes later I started to hum the Shania Twain song "Up," and I wondered why. My mind then went back to my trip to Victoria a couple months back, when the tour guide on the bus told us that Sidney, British Columbia, had the highest number of libraries per capital. I corrected myself: it's not library, it's book stores. I then noticed a small mall with a library. I continued on with my trip and noticed that I had passed my stop. When I finally got back to the address, I realized that the address that I was looking for was one stop after that library. The universe was trying to tell me that I must get off at the next stop, because the address is just "up" from here, like the song title.

I'm sure you are asking what this has to do with money. Well, I will tell you. I was 10 minutes late for the meeting. During the meeting with Gail, I told her that I really wanted to take the program; the only thing holding me back was finance. She then told me about funding available from the different government agencies for student loans and grants. While she was talking, I knew I would not be qualified for any of those programs. Instead, I realized that I could make a very good living by writing articles for a magazine or newspaper. Then Sarah Jessica Parker's character from the show *Sex and the City* popped into my head. It occurred to me that I would write articles in the same format as she did, with the topics being about weight management. This would allow me to study full-time and support myself by doing something that I love. I could write my story on a weekly basis and email it in. What I had to do was figure out how to find this magazine, newspaper, or TV with whom I would work.

Five days later, I started to have a recurring dream. On October 13, 2004, I dreamt that I was at work and had left the store unattended to get a cup of tea. I ran into Susan, one of my staff. At the coffee shop I ordered a cup of tea, and the server said, "You don't want mint tea?" I got extremely confused as to what I wanted. She then put a large cup of tea on the counter, and I picked it up. There was another female customer there who told me it was hers. I appeared confused again and gave it back, saying I thought it was wrong because it was a berry-red colour.

I got mine and went to the cake shop, where I bought an entire cake. The lady packed it up in a double-boiler pot, with the cake on the bottom and hot, steaming water on top to keep it warm. She told me that I must have the pot back to her by 5:00 p.m. I told her that it was already 4:45, but she said there were no exceptions. I said okay and left, walking through the mall and looking at the new store and the beautiful Sears window with several beautiful evening gowns.

Then I was walking outside, and I realized that I did not have the cake. I put my purse on the side of the road, which appeared to be a country road, and started running back to the cake store. I ran past a couple. The woman was very pale with long, straight black hair; she smiled at me and was happy with how I was running. I then saw a man with a brown purse picking up my black purse. I started to scream that it was my purse. He took off with the purse. I asked another man to help me chase the thief down, and we both took off. I caught up with the thief and jumped on him, and we fell to the ground. I then said, "Please give me my money back," and then I bit him on his chin. I told him that I had to pay my rent and bills, but I could give him $200 this week and $800 next week.

The second version happened on October 19, 2003, when I woke up that morning from a recurring dream. I dreamt that I opened my wallet, and there was a withdrawal slip from the bank stating that I withdrew $800 from my account. I was very confused and asked myself what I'd done with the money. I then realized that I'd used it to pay my rent. Later in the afternoon I had another dream that I was at work, and I told the staff that the visual technician would be in at 8:00 a.m. to remerchandise. I told them that I would be in between 8:30 and 9:00.

The following day when I got to work, I saw that the front section of the wall was done, and I told her it looked good. While making my way to the back of the store, I realized that nothing else was done. When I went to put my backpack into my locker, I realized that I had left my purse at home. I did not have money to buy lunch, and so I had to eat the granola bar and two chocolate bars in my backpack.

After both dreams of leaving my purse, I got a call from a staff member saying that I'd left my keys in the store. This led me to believe that leaving the store unattended and leaving my keys in the store was my subconscious mind telling me that I was to leave my current employer.

Confirmation of this happened on Tuesday, October 20, 2003, when I kept waking up and looking at the clock with anticipation. I could not wait to go to work, which I could not explain.

At work I took my lunch break at 1:30 p.m. After having my lunch, I decided to go out for a cup of tea. On my way I ran into a woman I recognized, but I could not recall her name. She said hello, and I asked her where I knew her from. She said she was Maddi, the manager from the maternity store in the mall. She asked how things were going, and I told her that business was very slow. She then told me that business in their company was booming, and she asked if I would be interested in joining her company. We exchanged phone numbers.

The following day her supervisor, Cheryl, called and made arrangements for an interview the next day. This meeting did not seem like an interview; rather it was a meeting to convince me to join the company. I felt great after the two-and-a-half-hour meeting, where Cheryl offered me $2000 above what I was making at my current company. I told her that I would have to check out the location before accepting her offer.

I called her that Monday and told her that the commute was fine but that it was an expensive bus ride. She then asked me whether I would accept if she gave me an extra $1000. I said yes, and she told me she needed authorization from the vice president. She called me back in an hour with the okay she needed. My conclusion of these events was that I was to leave my current employer, not go back to school, and continue my lessons in retail in another environment. When the time was right for me to attend college, the money would be there. I learned that the universe will give me not necessarily what I want, but what I need and what is in my best interests.

During my stay with this new organization, I met some wonderful friends and teachers who made it possible for me to learn and practice the very important lesson of forgiveness. I embraced my life lessons and teachers, and I became more at peace and comfortable with each area of my life, including my financial situation. I started to ask what I could do to remove this fear of abundance. Paying attention to the universe and its messages would alleviate my fears of accepting the gifts of the universe so that all of my needs of abundance will be met. Thoughts of money are messages from the universe for me to focus on my dreams. I believe that I will not be able to hold on to money until I learn how to share abundance with others who need it.

Ask yourself, "What is money preventing me from doing?" In my case, if I had all the money in the world, I would study wellness counselling in college full-time. This choice would allow me to live with purpose by studying, writing, and teaching weight management.

Leaving my last job was about spending the necessary time with myself in order to hear the guidance that I needed to walk my path. What does money have to do with my living on purpose? I was using lack of money for not moving on with purpose as an excuse to stay stuck. I repelled abundance because of the fear of my inner power, strength, and destiny. What is my emotional connection to money? It's an excuse for me not to follow my dreams of being a spiritual writer, speaker, counsellor coach, and healer. For me, money eases my mind so that I can concentrate on my craft of helping people who need it, whether or not they can afford it.

I must provide the service of the connection between nutritional, emotional wellness, living on purpose, and weight management to all women who need my assistance. I should give without expecting anything in return. Money makes me perform my work without worry. When I spend money on someone, it represents love and acceptance of who I am and what I do. By loving and accepting myself, I will love and accept others, and abundance of the universe will flow freely toward me for the use of helping.

Lately I have been very worried that I might miss the sign of abundance. My fears of abundance are raising their head again; this is the money that I am asking for to implement Healthea Solutions so that I can start helping women manage their weight. I am worried because sometimes I don't see the answers to my questions, because I don't recognize or accept the package in which it shows up. Healthea Solutions is the perfect way for me to help women because the business plan consists of all the things I love. It's my intention to make an excellent living doing what I love and helping others at the same time. It's possible that in the past I was not able to hold on to money because I did not earn it doing something I loved. I know how to make money doing what I don't like; now it's time to reverse that trend.

This fear disrupted my sleep. I kept waking up every

two hours and freaking out over my financial situation. I was confused as to what I was worried about because I was convinced that the money would be there for me at the appointed time. I then realized that it was not the money I was worried about; rather, it was my fear of what the universe was going to ask me to do for the cash—and the fear that I may not recognize it when it arrived.

I will recognize it like I recognize other things in the past, such as when I knew I had to move to Vancouver. All I need to do is trust and believe in my ability to know and recognize the truth when it shows up, regardless of its packaging. When the student is ready, the teacher will appear. When Althea is ready to receive, the cash will be visible. The following day I received an unexpected cheque to cover my rent that month. I now recognized one of my signs that I would be receiving money, and that was when I became overemotional about what I perceived as a lack of money. The universe is giving me the heads-up that money is coming my way.

Another example occurred on October 1, 2003. I woke up and wrote for about an hour. Later that morning while getting ready for my retail job, I realized that I was feeling extremely happy and excited. I told myself it must be because I had been writing earlier. I then said to God, "This is how I want to spend my time."

I started to daydream about what I would do if I won the lottery. I decided I would take all my fellow store managers out for lunch or dinner. I then thought to myself, *It's not about impressing others with your money. It's about showing them how to live a healthy and balanced life.* That could be through losing weight to improve health, personal development, career, financially, relationships, home, or spiritual development.

I came up with a great idea of contacting IHN (IHN is

the Institute of Holistic Nutrition, where I studied holistic nutrition and started my journey toward permanent weight management and mental, emotional, physical, and spiritual health and wellness) and setting up a scholarship program for those who needs financial support for education. The reason for this program is because I believe it's not right for someone to lose her home or independence just because she decides to go back to school. IHN is the Institute of Holistic Nutrition, where I studied holistic nutrition and started my journey toward permanent weight management and mental, emotional, physical, and spiritual health and wellness.

My relationship with IHN started after my mother's death, when I realized that I had to do something to save my life before I died at an early age like she did. I decided to start with my weight. I went to see a nutritionist whose number I had been sitting on for the past six months. After being a client of hers for about a year, I saw dramatic changes in my body, mind, and spirit. I then decided that I would love to help others to get to this point, so I pulled out the phone book and looked up nutritionists. I called several and asked where they went to school. I found out that this was not a licensed industry; however, there were accredited schools for those who would like to be formally educated. That was how I found IHN.

My money challenges taught me three things. The first was that it got me to understand how important it is for me to give to others that are less fortunate. How do I share my abundance with the universe? It's not about accumulating material possessions; it's about sharing what I have. I don't own things, I share things. The best way to receive love is to give back. Sharing is how I release and move the energy I am suppressing with food. It's not about making more money; it's about how to live on purpose, and how to give back by being. It's about taking without using up all that's available.

It's about giving of myself freely. It's also about accepting each person as she is without passing judgment. My money situation is not about Mom or my childhood; it's about acceptance, and giving and receiving without attachment. My challenges taught me that money does not make you a better person, friend, or daughter; it accentuates who you really are at your core.

Everything came together for me on Tuesday, June 1, 2004, when I was listening to Gary Zukav's book on tape, *The Mind of the Soul.* Zukav was telling the story of a preacher named Jonathon who spent years preaching against and condemning prostitutes. I recognized the story because I was and still am a fan of this preacher. I then asked myself what or whom have I been ignoring in my life. The answer was the relationship that I have with money and my friends.

All my friends, with the exception of Laurie, are either in the same financial situation as I am or worse. The one that I want to spend the most time with is Laurie. However, she is not open to a closer relationship with me, whereas others who are less fortunate want to spend more time with me. This is the universe's way of telling me that I am not ready for money. I will be ready when I realize that I have all the money I need, and more will show up when I truly need it.

I then went back into the next room to continue listening to the tape. Gary was recalling how he wrote his first book, *The Dancing Wu Li Masters.* I realized that I'd bought it years prior and had not read it. I then went to my bookcase, where the book was located behind an angel figure holding a basket. I picked up the angel, and several quarters fell to the floor; there was also a loonie in the angel's basket. I must have put them there for laundry and had forgotten about them. I was stunned and started to laugh when I realized the significance of this event. This is the universe telling me that I must change my ways and look for the good in mankind. This confirmed for me that when I become conscious, the money will be present, and my cups will runneth over with abundance.

Money is a metaphor for me to listen without judgment, to accept without judgment, and to accept the value in my and others' opinions. The universe is telling me that I have great instincts to follow, and I should trust them. I don't need money to follow my dreams; I just need to do what I love and what will make me happy, and the money will come. This quote says it all: "Every man is my superior in that I may learn from him." It also occurred to me that we make plans of how we would spend money if we got an inheritance or won the lottery. However, very few of us think of how much good we can do with this money to help others. What does this have to do with weight management, you may ask? It's not about giving money away; rather, it's about helping others who may need a hand up. It's about being of service.

There are millions of people in the world who are unhappy with their current situations. On one hand they know exactly where they would like to be. On the other hand they are afraid to leave their stable paycheque and go out on their own because of family obligations or the fear of failure. We do know that by following our truths, we will continue to manage our weight with little effort.

Donating our time, energy, and money to helping others in need is a great way to feed our souls. When our souls are fed, then we have no reason to binge on harmful foods that increase our weight and decrease our overall health. Giving money away is a win-win situation for the giver and the receiver, providing it's from the heart. Give because it's the right thing to do. Give without expecting something in return. Give because it feels good to give. It is within my power to share all that I have with others. With that said, it's not my concern what people do with the money; it is between them and God Almighty.

The Money-Weight Message

During a conversation with a friend, she recommended the book *Reinventing Your Life* by Jeffrey Young. It sounded amazing, so I called my nearby Chapters, who did not have it in stock but found it at another store. Instead of going downtown to pick it up, I decided to go to the library. On my way I said out loud to myself, "I hate getting books from the library because I prefer to buy them." Then I thought, *Oh well, you can't live in a book.* I then started to sing the Canadian national anthem; in fact, I could not stop singing it all the way to the library. I know—what a strange thing to do in that moment.

I got the book, and on my way home I recalled another thing that had happened during my conservation with my friend. She had mentioned that when she did not have money, she did not have to worry about eating foods that were unhealthy. Now that she had money, it was a concern. I then told her I recently discovered that food and money are two sides of the same coin. She agreed because they are both energy. I told her that I wanted to understand it, and we agreed to work on it together.

After recalling that conversation, I then started to sing the American national anthem. It was even more strange because I am a Canadian and only know the American anthem from watching sporting events on TV. I sang it all the way home—or should I say, I butchered it. As I was singing, I saw a young man sitting on the corner of the street, panhandling. I smiled at him, and while waiting for the light I opened my wallet and gave him a quarter, which was all I had.

These chains of events caused me to take a closer look at my thoughts, beliefs, and relationship with money. I realized that the singing of the Canadian national anthem and saying "You can't live in a book" was telling me that I was exchanging the energy of money for the knowledge in this book. I was being forced to look at my belief that if I borrowed it, I would have to give it back because it was not mine. On the other hand, if I bought it, then it belonged to me. The events reminded me that to learn, grow, and develop as an individual, I must share all that I am with others. Knowledge is free and should be shared. I discovered that I associated owning things with personal security. But I would always have knowledge when I needed it. Books for me were a fountain of knowledge, so buying a book meant its knowledge was for my own consumption. Borrowing meant it was to be shared with others. I could choose to share my knowledge of weight management with others, or I could selfishly keep it all to myself.

I've come to understand that my belief of what money is and what it does for me is misguided and limited. At the time I believed that money was comfort, that spending gave me energy, that spending made me feel strong and powerful, and that money gave me the opportunity to do what I loved without worry of survival. *Althea, are you saying that for you, money is survival?* No, despite all that money provides, it's just a temporary fix for a deeper problem, which is that I was using material possessions to try to be happy. I now know that the material possessions will not make me feel fulfiled and happy as long as I continue to eat to feel nourished, spend to feel safe and secure, eat to suppress, and spend to calm down.

Food and money are two sides of the same coin, and I

realized that to me food was all about self-indulgence, whereas money was about self-absorbance. What does all this mean? Well, the lack of money forced me to take a closer look at my life and how I was using it. Is it possible that those of us with money issues have issues because we are not using our lives to help others? In my case, I learned that when I am behind in my bills, I am on the wrong path, and I must take a step backward in order for me to focus on how I am following my destiny, which is to serve others and not myself. It's not about throwing money at others; it's about giving them my time. The only way I am going to maintain my weight is to help others with their own weight issues and lead them to fulfiled lives. That's a win-win situation for everyone involved.

When you are having money difficulties, ask yourself, "What am I really concerned about?" Then make a list and then evaluate your priorities. Look at what purpose these things serve in your life and whether or not you can live without them. Then look at how you can transfer this energy into helping another person. You will soon realize that the situation will improve when you set out to help others.

One day I was reminded of this fact when I woke up feeling sad about my financial situation. Even though it was raining, I decided to go for my regular morning walk. For the first time I could not concentrate on my surroundings; instead, I was overwhelmed with thoughts of my life. I realized that I was extremely disappointed, ashamed, and embarrassed with the state of my life. I was asking myself what I had done with my life, and the answer was nothing. I realized that I had not done anything of significance in the world. Here I was today, not knowing how I was going to pay my rent. I had no job, no husband, and no children. I had done nothing to help the world. I had contributed nothing to the betterment of the human race. It's not that I didn't want to help; it's that I was extremely confused and frustrated as to what I could do to help others. All this left me feeling extremely resentful at God and the universe. Here I was ready, willing, and able to help others, and all I had been experiencing were roadblocks every step of the way.

Instead of concentrating on finding a way to help, I was instead consumed with thoughts of how I was going to pay the rent. From where was the money to pay the bills going to come? Why did I continue to have money problems? What lesson was the universe trying to teach me with this lack of abundance?

I needed to switch my focus, my priority. Instead of being consumed with thoughts of lack in what I didn't have in career, money, and personal weight management, I must instead focus on what I did have: the skills to inspire women to make a change.

For some reason, at the time I could not get past thinking of myself and what I didn't have. I knew that my life purpose was to help others improve their health and to encourage personal development; however, there was no money to pay the bills so that I could concentrate on making it a reality. No matter where I turned, the door was closed to me. I decided to put that goal on hold and instead look for a job doing something similar. I had the same results as before: no one was hiring.

I now believe that the reason why I have been having difficulty funding my career is that I was placing my focus on *me* and what I want, instead of being of service to others. I was focusing on lack, which resulted in lack expanding and magnifying in my life. I now understand that by helping someone to make a personal change, I will automatically see a change in my own personal circumstances. To attract the financial capital needed, I must focus on the end result, which is what I intend to use this capital for: being of service to women on their weight management journeys.

"As you think, so you become; as you become, so you see how you have been thinking" is one of my favourite quotes. Focusing on being of service will always lead you in the right direction. Putting your attention on what you don't have will bring you more of what you don't want, resulting in increased appetite and excessive weight gain.

I had a quest to answer all-important questions: "What can I do today to achieve success? What can I do to attract more money? What lesson am I to learn from putting my goals on hold, leaving behind the very things that I believe will make me truly happy at last?" I have learned that the energy that is money is telling me that I have not been following the signs of the universe, which have been telling me that I am channelling my energy in the wrong direction.

All my plans have been about self-improvements from a materialistic, self-centreed point of view, instead of from a holistic viewpoint that incorporates the wants and needs of others. These are the things that would make me look great in the eyes of the world. From the outside looking in, the package is beautiful, whereas on the inside it is dying from a lack of nurturing. It's about learning what parts of me are wounded so that they can be healed.

I came to the realization that we are all born wounded in some form, with two goals in mind: identify and admit to being wounded, and find someone with the same issues and help them work through it. You need a partner to do this because it's not possible to heal it in yourself; you can't see it as clearly in yourself. You need to find others with the same wound so that you can heal it in them and within yourself at the same time.

I've come to understand that having money to carry out

the list above would not make me happy, because it's a front; in fact, I would end up in the same position as before within a year, which is feeling that there is more to life than what I am doing. It's the feeling that I need to help others in a meaningful way by helping them grow. It's about finding the root cause of unhappiness, to which the symptom is financial worry.

With all that being said, we need to ask ourselves whether this is the right time, condition, and place to carry out this dream. We need to look at the time frame, condition, and place when thinking of changing direction in life, because there is a season for all things, and it's quite possible that one or a combination of all will be out of sequence. It's about listening to the universal signs, which will tell us when it's okay to carry out our life purposes and destinies at the right time and place, and under the right conditions. We must to do what we love in accordance with our true destinies.

It's also a message for us to go after the sustenance of life instead of the frills, which will result in happiness and fulfilment. No amount of money can fill up that empty space inside of us that is desperately looking for love, acceptance, and guidance—the little child that is desperately searching for a way to help others who need it. My discontent was about me wanting to do the right thing, but I didn't know what that was, so I got angry and frustrated and acted by hurting myself by overeating and overspending,

Lack of money is telling me that the right time, place, or conditions for my dream to come true are missing. The dream is to have financial stability so that I can carry out the action plan of helping others improve their health and personal development.

When time is the issue, then the message is telling me that the lack of money is a sign for me to slow down. It's a way of keeping me from moving forward too quickly, and for me to think before leaping without all the information I need in order to be successful. Stop rushing through your life. If you continue to rush, then you will miss your guidance and the life lessons. The learning is in the present moment, the here and now.

When place is the issue, the universe is telling me that money can only help shape my destiny, but it's not the destiny. I learned this over the years when I noticed that when I was living in accordance with the universe, I could save money and everything was going great. On the other hand, when I was on the wrong track, I seemed to have money difficulties. Lack of money is a sign for me to stop and take a closer look at what direction I am heading in. I should look back and identify the signs that I was heading in the wrong direction.

For example, when I received guidance to finish school and move back to Toronto, the guidance did not mention which school—was it Rhodes Collage or Naropa University? Where I moved to next would determine where I set up Healthea Solutions. I choose to have a condo in Toronto and attend Naropa University for the next four years while working part-time with Healthea Solutions. Now, that was my goal, but it did not necessarily mean that this was my destiny. I was prepared to adjust it by making changes, whether great or small. I was also prepared to completely abandon these three ideas and follow another path. It was entirely up to the universe; I was the vessel delivering the message, but I was not the message. *What about deciding to go back to school for a year without working?*

When the issue is the conditions, the lack of money is trying to get me to stop rushing and take stock of what I am doing, thinking, and feeling regarding my purpose and direction in life. Lack of money is all about giving my energy away, misplacing it, and dropping the ball. It's telling me that I need to focus on what I do have instead of what I don't have, which will in turn open the door for other things.

This is the perfect opportunity to look at and come to an understanding of the emotions behind my relationship with money, because making money doing what I live does not change my money problems, which is my feelings about money. Once I make money, what do I do with it? What are the emotions behind my relationship with money?

Money that is needed to carry out purpose and destiny will be manifested with the understanding of emotions behind the giving and receiving of money. I now know that the lack of financial support is a message to stop and take stock of my life's direction. I am being given the opportunity to look within in order to learn something new, or to receive the answer that I have been searching for, without interference from the outside world. I now see my lack of control and direction with my career, money, and weight management, and it has taught me to take this opportunity to channel my energy into another direction, to look at these challenges as an opportunity to look and feel different, to change how I view the world and my contribution to it.

More important than money is personal satisfaction in what I do! I now view money as a vehicle that creates movement, transporting me where I need to go in order to do the most good. By spending money on junk, I'm telling the universe where I want to go. So it's not about dieting. It's about moving, changing, and shifting; it's about the healing of the mind, body, and spirit. When we are happy with how we are making a living, then we tend to use our money wisely. We invest our money in people and things we enjoy.

WEIGHT AND RELATIONSHIPS

What constitutes a relationship? A relationship is being connected to someone or something else. It's the deep, spiritual connection you have with yourself and with the people, places, and things around you. This includes your spouse, parents, siblings, friends, acquaintances, employer, and coworkers.

All relationships start with our mothers, fathers, and other caregivers. How we were treated as infants is reflected in how we treat others and ourselves today. If they were loving and patient with us, then we will be loving and patient with ourselves. If they ignored our feelings, then we will ignore our own emotions. We mirror our parents' behaviours because that's what we were taught. It's what we know. The same tool they use to keep us out of their way as a child is what we use today to avoid making a decision, taking action, and moving forward in life. We are simply perpetuating what we learned while growing up. How many times did you say you would not do the same things that your parents did—only to see and hear yourself doing and saying those same things? That's not a coincidence; we are doomed to repeat what we've seen and heard until we wake up and make a conscious choice to change that behaviour.

As a result, we become overweight because our relationship with a part of our life needs healing. Is it our relationship with our parents, ourselves, or food? All this leads to an imbalance in our career, finances, health and fitness, relationships, home, personal growth and development, and spirituality.

Numerous books have been written on relationships over the years. What it comes down to is having the right group of people around you who will help you live a happy and fulfiled life. These people are uniquely suited to you. My intention is to get you to take a closer look at the people in your life currently, focusing on these questions:

- Who are they?
- What's their purpose in your life?
- What are you to learn from them?
- What are you to teach them?
- How open are you to these lessons and teachers?

With that in mind, let's examine the different types of relationships and the purpose of each in your life.

Self

Your connection with yourself is the most important relationship you have. Know that you are perfect as you are, regardless of your dress size. Know that the excess weight you are carrying around does not define who you really are; this weight is a teacher designed to get you focusing on you and your own personal wants, needs, and desires. The excess fat is telling you that you are out of balance and off track in certain parts of your life. By focusing on your own health, you will find the truth and your way back on track.

Your relationship with yourself always starts with the

decision in knowing what or who is best for you. Are you with this person, place, or thing because you want to be, or is it out of guilt and or obligation? Making the decision to be with him or her because it's what you want and need is respecting yourself. It's for your greater good.

The ultimate relationship with the self is to know who you truly are at the core; it's having the awareness of the essence of your authentic self. A strong, healthy relationship with the self involves being honest and true to what you need and desire. It's loving yourself enough to say no to toxic relationships. Instead, you build and nurture strong, healthy relationships with others. In the end it will make you stronger. I'm doing a disservice to the other person and myself each time I say yes when I don't want to do it. It's robbing us both of a great relationship with someone else we both deserve.

The perfect relationship with the self involves loving and respecting yourself for who you are and what you are, regardless of what others may say or think. It's your life to live the way that's most comfortable for you.

I learned this the hard way. Until I was 5 years old, I spent all my waking moments with my maternal grandfather, who made me feel very loved and safe. Then he died, and my whole world changed. After the funeral, my family continued on as before. However, I had just lost the love of my life, and I now found myself alone literally and figuratively. I did not have Papa to talk to, and everyone else was too busy to talk to me.

This left me feeling very angry in my adult years. As a way to control this anger, I turned to food to soothe my feelings. For many years I was unaware of this anger. Once I was aware of it, I could not understand from where this anger came. I knew that my family loved me, and they always made sure I was clothed and fed, so why was I so angry?

I was angry because I wanted them to take the time to listen to me the way Papa did. Having material things was great, but I put more value in being seen, heard, and acknowledged. I've come to understand that the lesson was being comfortable with being by myself to replenish my energy. This includes learning to stand alone when necessary. Part of self-care is taking time for yourself and by yourself. It also involves being consciously aware of unexpressed or unresolved emotions, feelings, behaviours, attitudes, wants, needs, and desires.

Self-intimacy means knowing yourself on a deeper spiritual and soul level. It's when you dig deep within your own mind. Body. and spirit for the purpose of knowing your true nature, needs, and desires. It's knowing what truly makes you feel content and fulfiled.

Romance

I am using the word "spouse" in a traditional way because that's what it means to me: a married man and woman who have pledged partnership with each other. In today's society the word "spouse" means different things to different people. In some cases it's in the form of a same-sex couple. It can also be in the form of a common-law arrangement. Regardless of what label you put on it, it's the same, so you can feel free to use whatever term that's most comfortable to you. When I was growing up, family and friends used such terms as "my other half," "the old man," "the little woman," "my mate," and "my significant other."

A spousal relationship is a balancing act between being an individual and a couple. Being in a relationship is part of the human experience. It's being in a deep, intimate relationship with another person. It's about sharing your mind, body, and spirit with another. It's sharing your most inner-most thoughts, feelings, beliefs, ideas, needs, and desires. It's having someone in your life that is always, and you support each other in all facets of life.

To me, having a spouse is having a best friend, companion, lover, and confidant all in one package. This is the person I rely on and trust most; it's with whom I want to make a family. Some people refer to this person as a soul mate.

A spousal relationship teaches us how to be one of or part of, and how to be connected to another person while maintaining our individuality. It's putting what we have learned from our parents into action. It's about building a life with someone else and forming a family.

How does this type of relationship affect your weight? When you are in a loving, passionate, and committed relationship, where you love and are loved by another in an intimate way, then you will eat small, healthy meals for fuel. If you feel repressed, then you will lose or gain weight when you start to realize that it's not the relationship you are seeking.

The excessive weight gain begins when we give our power to our spouses. We are willingly expecting them to take over our life from where our parents left off. In my case, I was looking for someone to take care of me, to give me the love and support that was missing since the death of my grandfather. I want someone who sees, hears, knows, recognize me for who I am and the work I do, and who showers me with an abundance of love and affection.

With all that said, was I longing for a husband or for a parent? Looking back on my past romances, I realize why they did not last. I was looking to them for the love I did not receive from my family while I was growing up.

What I've learned over the years is that there is no one on

earth that can give that to me—except me. As much as I say I'm tired of being alone and taking care of myself, I finally admitted to myself that though I'm angry about not being loved the way I wanted to be loved as a child, I must get over it. This attitude is keeping me away from true, authentic romance. I must decide once and for all what I want and then do it for myself. Once I start being my own parent, then I automatically attract others who want to be there for me without ulterior motives.

I realized that this longing to be taken care of was leftover trauma from my childhood. As a child I came home to an empty house because my grandmother was at work, my grandfather was dead, and my uncles were out living their own lives. As a result, today I find it difficult to come home to my beautiful apartment because I live alone. I'm longing for the day when I will come home to someone who loves and cares about me. As far back as I can remember, I can only recall a handful of times I came home and there was a family member waiting for me. It's not that I love being alone; it's that I don't have a choice in the matter. After Papa died, my uncles and grandmother were busy. There was little time for me. Oftentimes Mama told me to go to the neighbours when it got dark. Today I don't know where to go when it gets dark, so I stay home, eat, and watch television. Do I do this because I feel safe or unsafe? Or is it simply out of habit?

I've come to understand that I can choose to be lonely, or I can choose to be with others, even if I find them boring. The thing is that they are not the boring ones—I'm simply bored with myself and am transferring these feelings onto them! I'm feeling this way because I'm tired of doing the same thing day in and day out. I must change my actions; however, for some reason I'm not willing to do so. It's not about being lonely; it's about wanting more from myself. I have a great home and a fantastic life, and my soul is reminding me that I must share it with someone else.

What this journey has taught me is to really look at my actions. When all is said and done, the bottom line is that I must take responsibility for my own personal needs and desires. I must decide what I want and go after it. I have to stop looking for someone to take care of me and do it myself with lots of love. What I do need is someone with whom to share my life. I don't need a parent—I need a husband.

Is it your intention to ground yourself, to settle down in one spot with one person? Then marriage is for you. If you need to run free, then the opposite is true for you. Always be honest with yourself. I have a lot going on and would love someone with whom to experience it. What it comes down to is that I have lots of great females in my life, but what I really want and need is a husband.

Friendships

What is friendship? According to the dictionary definition, it's a type of relationship between two people who care about each other. For me, it's about two or more people with shared interests, goals, and backgrounds getting together and having a good time. It's a group of people uplifting each other in a positive way. And then there are those people who seem to think friendships are for dumping their problems; I call these people energy vampires.

I have several great female friends in my life today, and yet I feel very much alone. It took me awhile to figure out that I'm not a huge fan of typical friendships. There are some who believe that talking every day is what friendships are all about. I've often wondered what on earth I possibly have to say to the same friend each day. Based on my personal beliefs, it sounds like checking in with a counsellor, and this kind of relationship does not appeal to me. I just want to go out and have a good time with my friends, not counsel them.

I find that most of my friends these days are calling me crying about their struggles. Coaching and counselling is what I absolutely love to do; however, when I come home after work, I want to relax and have a little fun. In a way my friends' complaining was tainting my relationship with the work I loved to do. Dealing with emotional issues on a daily basic is draining, and if I'm not careful, I will burn out. That's one of the reasons I want to leave my work at the office. Coming home gives me the opportunity to recharge my batteries, which makes me a balanced and better coach.

One day I found myself ignoring the calls from a couple of my closest friends, and I started to examine my reaction. That's when I realized that I find our interactions with each other extremely draining. I noticed that after I got off the phone with them, I was so drained myself that I would go straight to the kitchen for something to eat, as a way of increasing my energy level. I realized that they were calling me at all times of the day and night, upset about their various life challenges. I would always take their calls because I really wanted to help them.

I started asking myself probing question to understand my motives. "Is it possible that I'm avoiding them because I'm avoiding and resisting my gift of helping women heal in mind, body, and spirit? Yes! I'm resisting Healthea Solutions Weight Management and Wellness Centre!"

These women are fantastic gifts who have helped me to own and accept my faith as a weight management coach, motivational speaker, and counsellor. My being overweight is a clear indication that I was resisting my true calling, my true destiny. My abdominal area is my career, my life purpose, what I'm here to help others with. And there lies my friendship dilemma. I like and want to spend time with them—I just don't want to be their personal counsellor. I want to keep my work and personal life separate. Why do I continue to attract these women who are energy vampires? What am I to learn from these experiences? There are life lessons: setting clear boundaries, accepting my gifts, and being true to myself.

I'm manifesting what I've been thinking about, and they are here to remind me to look at my challenges. What I'm lacking are clear boundaries of when I'm to help versus when I'm to take time for myself. I love helping women with their emotional issues, but I don't want to mix business with pleasure. What are boundaries? They are specific sets of personal guidelines outlining rules and limits of what one finds acceptable. It's telling and showing others how to treat us.

The second part of the attraction to energy vampires is for the sole purpose of owning and accepting my gift as a healer. It's interesting that I was looking for people who are fun loving, for people who are not trapped within their own pain. I was attracting these people for two reasons: they're telling me that I do have the gift for helping them get out of their current circumstances, and that I'm stuck in my own pain and must address it. I'm turning to food because the latter part is the most dominant reason why I'm attracting this type of friend; as long as I'm eating and burying my pain, I don't have to address it.

So what does all this have to do with friendships? For most of my life I've been a loner, which most people don't understand. It's simple, really: I work all day with people who are constantly pulling at me, constantly asking for this, that, and everything. At times it becomes overwhelming. This leaves me feeling angry and frustrated because I feel I can't finish what

I've started. I have a long list of things to do and am unable to accomplish them because someone always interrupts me. For me, solitude is all about recharging my battery. It's about having peace of mind.

How does the types of friends I keep contribute to my weight gain and losses? I must give myself what I need. It's okay for me to ask for and take the time I need for myself so that I can replenish my energy. I'm turning to food because I'm angry at myself for not giving myself what I need in the moment. I must give myself permission to take care of myself before I can help others.

The next time the phone rings, will you look at the displayed number and get excited, or do you immediately think, *Good grief, what's wrong this time?* Being happy about the call is a clear indication of the joy this person brings to your life. On the other hand, feeling that you have to take the call even though you don't want to is telling you that you are not interested in anything this person has to say. In fact, you are only taking this call out of obligation to the past.

It's time to look within and get extremely real with yourself about your current behaviour. You are not happy about getting the call because you are not willing to look at your own behaviours, feelings, and thoughts. Each time you are tempted to ignore seeing or talking to someone, ask yourself, "What am I not ready to face at this time? Why is that am I not ready to accept this about myself? What's the worst that can happen if I face this truth today? What gifts might I receive from this circumstance? What is this relationship saying about me? They are forcing me to look at a part of my life that I don't care to examine at this time. What's the fear about? What is it about relationships that scare me? I don't like people to get too close to me—why? It then becomes about their wants needs and desires instead of mine. It's my need to be acknowledged."

There are some friendships that I find extremely overbearing. I feel this way not because of them; instead it's how I'm feeling about me. I find most of my female friends to be very needy, which I find annoying. The only female friends I want around me are happy, fun-loving people who bring out the same thing in me.

Today I'm surrounded by lots of unhappy people who bring out the anger in me. I do know it's their role in my life—showing me my pain and anger, exposing my pain so that I have the opportunity to clean and heal the wound. They are loving teachers showing me the way of healing so that I can move on. They are exposing my hidden behaviours, thoughts, and feelings regarding where I want to be, what I want to do, and with whom I want to do it. I'm not taking their calls out of obligation; rather, I'm taking them because I'm willing to know, understand, and accept that angry, pissed-off, and frustrated part of me. There is a lesson there that I'm willing to learn today.

The trust factor is another component of a balanced friendship. How much do you trust the people in your life today? Do you trust them to keep your secrets, your inner-most feelings and desires? Will they keep what you have just shared, or will they tell their other friends?

While I was growing up, on several occasions my mother told us we didn't need female friends; whatever we told them would be gossiped about, and the whole world would know our business. It's not about being ashamed—it's about being private with our lives. The struggle now is that I don't want to share things with the people that are in my life today. I'm always saying, "I wish I had someone to talk to," but I do have lots of people who would be happy to listen to me vent. So why don't I want to let them in? The people who are close to me are in so much pain. How can I ask them to help me when they can't seem to help themselves? They have their own challenges they have to take care of before they can help me.

It's because I'm sitting back and waiting for others to stimulate me. I must make a list of events I'd like to attend and then go. It's like when I was a child waiting for someone to come home and take care of me. Simply put, I must take responsibility for my own happiness, my own excitement.

The next step in looking at the friendships in your life today is asking yourself, "Are they people I really want to be around? Do I enjoy being around them in the good and not-so-good times?" If they don't bring you joy, then it's time to grow up, find new friends, and be the leader of your own destiny. It's about doing what you love. If you're feeling bored, then you have no business being there or doing that.

I have a lot of wonderful and terrific friends whom I love very much. However, there was a time when I did not like some of them very much. During that time of my life, I found them to be extremely needy, wanting more and more of my time. At the time I felt I was giving them so much of myself that I did not have anything left to give myself. It's not about what they don't have or bring to the table; it's what I need.

There are three kinds of people in my life. The first kind are the fun-loving, passionate, warm, and exciting people whom I enjoy being around in good times and bad times. They are the ones who live each moment. They are present and focused in a strong, passionate way. When an issue arises in their lives, they deal with it in the moment. They know their past challenges, but they don't dwell on them. In fact, they look at each situation as a lesson to be learned. They hold nothing back and sometimes ask for help in moving on, without dwelling on the past.

The second people only show up just in time to teach me a valuable lesson. Sometime I help them, and other times they only show up to help me heal a situation I'm dealing with at that exact moment in time. It's interesting that I don't see them very often, and yet when we get together, it's as if we were never apart. We always end up helping each other tremendously.

The third group of people are those I always seem to attract in my personal life: the energy vampires. I love them in my working life but not in my personal life. They seem to drain my energy personally, whereas professionally they excite ne and give me more energy. They are people that I don't like being around personally and love professionally. Personally, the only reasons I speak or see them is out of obligation, because I feel I owe them something. I must move them from my personal life completely. I feel that their toxic energy is too much for me to deal with outside of work because they take up too much of my down time. In fact, I feel that I don't see the upside to having them in my personal life because all they do is drain my energy. Personally I just want to eat to drown them out, and professionally I'm so excited working with them that I forget to eat when around them. I do know firsthand that being alone is difficult; however, it's extremely unhealthy to be in an unfulfiling relationship. We should surround ourselves with people who increase instead of drain our energy. We then attract more like-minded people into our lives.

Over the past 30 years, I've come to understand that friendships also include learning how to support and be supported during each phase of life. Please realize that people enter our lives for the long-term and short-term, mirroring our own personal thoughts, feelings, beliefs, and ideas. They are showing me how I've been acting. Once I acknowledge these behaviours in myself, I will know exactly how to eliminate them in myself.

Acquaintances

Acquaintances are people who show up just in time, for a specific lesson and for a short period of time. They show us our behaviours so that we will know when we are on or off track, and they show us the way to get back on track. Most of the time, they are the most annoying people whom we can't seem to shake. Everywhere we go, there they are.

In my case, it's one specific group of people whom I will not name because their race is irrelevant. The lesson they have to teach me is all that matters. Let me start by telling you that I grew up in a neighbourhood where there was representation of every race and religion known to man. I was very comfortable with each and every one of them. Then I went away to college in the big city. This was the first time I was faced with large groups of various minority groups, including my own. I was shocked to see how segregated they were. I was raised with 90 percent Caucasian and 10 percent of all other races, but everyone got along. Meeting people who chose to segregate themselves was shocking, to say the least. I'm all for keeping up with traditions, but there are lots to be learned from others around us. For me, mingling is all about learning and expanding my horizon.

Then I started to realize that there was one group I found particularly offensive. I felt that they were the loudest and most obnoxious group of people. I found that most of them chose not to learn or speak English. I did not understand this, because why on earth did they fight so hard to get into this country and yet refuse to communicate with others who came before them?

In trying to communicate with them, I found that they were not interested. The only group of people they were interested in communicating with was themselves. Case in point: I went to a restaurant where there was a sign saying, "Wait to be seated." I stood there for 10 minutes, and no one came to seat me, so I left. When I told an employee of mine who was of the same race about the incident, she said, "You can't go by yourself—one of us has to be with you." I was shocked.

More and more I started to meet others of various races who felt the same way I did. In fact, most people from the other races felt this way. One day I went to a store to purchase vitamins, and the sales associate asked me where I was from. When I told her, she said she could not live there because of the large amounts of this group of people. I tried to leave several times, but she would not let me leave—she went on to tell me all the reasons she did not like them. Even though I did not want to have this conversation with her, I agreed with every word she said.

After being in retail for as long as I have been, my disdain for them had grown even more, so I believed that they were the problem. Then one day I asked myself, "Why do they ignore me when I say hello? Is it possible that they're ignoring me because they can sense my negative energy? They can feel that I don't really want to talk to them. They are indeed picking up on and mirroring my attitude." It then occurred to me that what I was projecting outward was what I was getting back.

I realized I must change my way of thinking of those I accuse of being a pain in my ass. In the past I simply walked away from them without addressing where these feelings were coming from. Leaving was not the answer because the problem was within me and would continue to travel with me.

Acquaintances are telling us that in order to teach, we must first become students. And so the story begins. It's about us understanding what makes us do the things we do and then using this newfound knowledge to help others heal. Experience, learn, teach!

I believe I can continually dwell on the past, or I can use my experience to help others. I believe that issues with my upbringing, weight, career, and finances are a road map for helping others heal. It's a lesson in knowing my truth and using this truth to help others and myself heal in mind, body, and spirit.

I don't like to be ignored, and I get angry at people who I feel are ignoring me. However, is it possible at they are ignoring me because I'm ignoring myself, and they are here to remind me of this fact? That's the perfect time to ask, "What truth must I acknowledge, accept, and recognize in myself?" These annoying people are my teachers who are here to get me back on track, and as soon as I'm back on track, they are then out of my life. The perfect example is Tonya. She hired me in Victoria and was extremely pleased with my work. In a very short period of time, I managed to staff the store and got it running smoothly. Then she convinced me to move to Langley because that store also needed help and had a higher volume of customers. Within a few months she was no longer happy with my work; I found this out on my review. Not once before my review did she tell me she was unhappy with my work. It took a year and a half for me to realize that she was in my life to get me back to the mainland. I was very happy being on the island, and I only left because of her. So why did I need to move back to Vancouver? I do love the city for its beauty and its closeness to the mountains and beaches. I feel very much at home in the city, and now I realize that it's where my soul belongs.

What am I to do in Vancouver that I could not do in Oshawa,

Pickering, North York, East York, Toronto, Burnaby, Victoria, or Langley? I needed to be in those places so that I could be certain that Vancouver is where I belong. Everything I do need in life to feel happy, fulfiled, and successful is in Vancouver. Vancouver is the one place that I can honestly say provides me with the balance I need in my life. I have the perfect amount of time spent at work and at play. That's what Gymboree has taught me. I do work hard and must take time to rest and relax so that I can replenish my energy. The same goes with family and friends: it's giving them time and also taking time for myself to replenish my energy. It's about balance.

With that said, why am I still overweight? Althea, it's about living on purpose. It's about developing and growing the Healthea Solutions Weight Management and Wellness Centre. I'm still unclear as to why I'm still overweight despite being in my ideal city. I must bring more balance into my career. I do spend a lot of time working to pay the bills; now it's time to put more energy into building my business. I should take more time to travel, study, write, and teach for the purpose of building Healthea Solutions Weight Management and Wellness.

You are putting on weight because you are ignoring the message. What message is that? To move on to something else. It's time for another change! What is it? I'm not interested in conversing with them because I just don't have anything to say on the matter. We might not like them, but their job is to show us what's missing and then direct us in the right direction to achieve success. They are here forcing me to acknowledge my anger at myself, and they're bringing out all I've been suppressing with food. The more I try to suppress, the angrier I become, and the more they will show up in my life. They help me to focus on the following aspects of my life:

- where I want to be
- what I want to do
- with whom I want to do it

Working Relationships

The average person does not have any say in with whom she works; the manager or owner of the company does. So, what do you do when you have to work with someone whose work ethic is not compatible with yours on the surface? What if it's the organization itself that you have a problem with? The way I see it, you have two choices: leave and go to another organization, or look within and learn the lesson being offered.

Over the first 25-plus years of my career, I would get so angry with the way a company was operating that I would quit and move to another company. I told myself that they didn't know what they were doing, despite the fact that all of them had been around for many years before I joined them.

I was working for a large Canadian retailer for two years when I started to question what was going on with my career. I realized it was not where I wanted to be, and that was why I was criticizing the company. This was abundantly clear the day the owner and president of the company announced that he was coming for a store visit. I was extremely angry. Why was I so angry? Store visits happened several times each year in every retail store I'd ever worked. This time the difference was the fact that he was coming on Thanksgiving Day. As a store manager, I was on salary and did not get overtime. All hourly employees got paid for the day plus time and a half if they worked it. For me, it counted as a regular day, so I'd always taken it off. To make matters worse, I had to work the Sunday as well to prepare for the visit, so there went my long weekend.

The closer we got to the visit, the angrier I became. As a result, I could not raise my left hand above my shoulder without experiencing excruciating pain. I'm not a doctor, but I attributed this intense pain to my anger. I was internalizing my rage, and it manifested itself in this manner. I felt stuck because I needed this job to cover my living expenses. As a single person, I had no one on whom I could lean financially, so I was stuck.

When he arrived for the visit, I was at the store's front greeting customers. He came in and, without saying hello, proceeded to ask why sales were down for the sister store next door. I told him I did not know, and my only interaction was when they had questions to help out because they didn't have a store manager. He did not acknowledge the fact that it was thanksgiving, and this made me even angrier. Despite my feelings toward him, I put on a brave face and continued with the visit. We went through the entire visit, and he was pleased with the store's sales appearance, the staff, and me.

One week after the visit, I was still angry. I was walking in the mall when I ran into a manager from another retailer in the mall. I recognized her because two weeks prior she was in my store trying to recruit me. She asked me how things were going, and I hesitated and then said okay. She then told me if I was looking for a change, her district manager would be in town the following day. I told her I had an appointment at 1:00 p.m., so if we could talk in the morning, it would be okay.

I met with the district manager on Thursday and had the most amazing three-hour interview that did not feel like an interview. She then offered me a job, and I accepted it three days later after some negotiation on my part.

As it turned out, I did not like this new company any better. I loved my employees and my district manager, but not the company. What a shocker. I started to wonder why everywhere

I went, it was usually the same: I get annoyed at the company I'm working for, and then leave, only to walk into a similar situation.

I am very good at what I do based on the results in sales and employee satisfaction, and yet I am not happy. Why? What's wrong? What am I looking for? What's missing? How many companies must I go through before I accept the fact that the problem lies within me?

After asking myself and answering the tough questions, I realized that it was not the companies—it was me. I was extremely angry at myself for being an employee instead of an employer. I wanted to work less and make more money. I've always wanted to be self-employed. As a result I was feeling trapped in the cycle, moving from one retail company to the next with the same result. Isn't that the definition of insanity?

I was longing to be my own boss, to be the one setting policies instead of enforcing them. It's interesting to look back at the last few companies I've worked for. I realize that with each new company, I was always working harder and harder, which was the opposite of what I wanted.

What do you do when the philosophy is dramatically different? What I've learned is that it's their company, which means they get to make the rules. If I want to make the rules, then I must have my own company. I've learned that the fastest way to be happy is staying put long enough to learn the lesson being offered. In times of difficulty, you can leave and start all over again, or you can simply ask, "What lesson am I to learn from this person or event?"

The relationship I was having with myself at the time was being reflected back at me through these wonderful organizations. There is an old saying, "No matter where I go, there I am." Just like me, if you are moving from place to place with the same unhappy outcome, then it's not the people, places, or events that are the issue. Instead, look within because that's where it's coming from. True happiness is in the learning and understanding your life challenges.

These organizations have showed me that I can follow their lead, living from paycheque to paycheque and being angry at the world for doing what they do best—or I can blaze my own trail to success. Sometimes I must follow, but for the most part I am a leader and must lead.

Our relationships teach us how to be a student in learning and how to take directions. They show us how to lead and teach what we know, as well as where to go in accessing the information needed for the next step in our journeys.

Family Dynamics

My family dynamic is very interesting. Let's start by saying I do have two different and distinct families that I refer to as my primary and secondary families. My first family consists of my maternal grandmother, grandfather, and two uncles, Ed and Ken. I was with most of them for the first 12 years of my life.

Why was I living with them? My mother gave birth to me at 18, out of wedlock. Back in the day, this did not happen. Despite the shame it brought on my family, I felt loved, wanted, and accepted by everyone involved. It was Mom's issues, not mine; I was not to blame for my mother's choices. It was also widely accepted that the grandparents take in the first grandchild if all parties agree. The idea was for this grandchild to take care of the grandparents in their golden years.

For the first five years I was the happiest child in the world. Every memory I have of Papa (my grandfather) involves me laughing and having a good time. He entertained me by taking walks with me, and while I was standing on his foot, he would hold my hands so that I could swing. Most important, he would listen to what I had to say; no matter how bizarre my questions, he would always give me an answer.

My first association with food being pleasurable (love) was with Papa. When he wanted to give me candy, he would unwrap it, put it between his lips, and then put his lips to mine and transfer the hard candy to my mouth. Even thinking about it 45 years later, it brings back the memory of pure joy. Wow, that was an amazing experience, being loved the way he loved and took great care of me.

Then it happened. Without warning he died, and I lost my best friend, caregiver, and confidant. There was no discussion of why he died, leaving me to wonder what I was to do now. He was buried in a tomb on the property, so when no one was looking I would go down there and play on his grave. When a family member would catch me there, the person would scold me and tell me that it was not a place for a child to play.

They were afraid that Papa's spirit would miss me so much that he would come back for me; that was why my favourite doll was buried with him. The thinking was that he would be forced to play with the doll, which would take my place in his heart. It's interesting that no one thought of giving me something to take his place in *my* heart—not that anyone or anything could have.

I was 6 years old and alone because Papa was dead, Mama (grandmother) was at work, and my two uncles, who were 10 and 12 years older than me, were busy living their lives. Most of the time Mama would tell me to go to my godfather's house when it got dark, if no one was home with me.

My second association of connecting food to love came from Mama. She worked for the minister of agriculture and often worked late. She would send dinner home for me with one of her coworkers. At 6 years old I came to the conclusion that this food was the next best thing to her love and attention.

Then at 12 years old Mama died, and I went to live with my other family. My second family is my biological mother, stepfather, two half-brothers, and two half-sisters. I love them very much. After Mama died, Mom thought it was time for me to live with them, so I did. I want to start off by saying that they are great people. The problem was I was an only child for the first 12 years of my life, and all of a sudden I had four siblings younger than me, and I had to help take care of them. I was extremely depressed due to the fact that I was living with strangers. They were my family, and so I had no choice but to do as I was told.

I was afraid to speak up because I did not want to be kicked out of the house for disobeying them. I felt trapped with no one to turn to for help and support. For years I suppressed my feelings with chocolate bars, sour cream and onion chips, French fries with gravy, pop, and other junk foods. I hid all that I felt I could not say. With each bite of food, I was also mourning my original family. I no longer felt safe and secure in this world. Despite living in a house full of people, I felt I had no one to whom I could talk. To make matters worse, I felt I had to compete with my siblings for our parents' attention and affection. I refused to do so and kept to myself most of the time.

I got the reputation for being quiet as a mouse. I also did not want to play games of competition. I wanted to be acknowledged for being a good person, for being me. In this family I felt trapped; there was no one to talk to and nowhere to go, so I kept doing what I was told, hating every second of it.

Then I discovered reading, and it saved my sanity. I started using my allowance to buy horror novels at the used book store.

When I was not doing chores, I always had my head in a book. This worked because Mom holds education in high regard. I was reading two books plus what I needed to read for school each week, and I loved it. During the summer I read four to five books weekly.

Mom and Stepfather made sure the fridge was always full with food. They worked extremely hard to put food on the table and a roof over our heads; to them, that was love. When I went away to college and would come back home for the holidays, Mom would make sure all my favourites were there. They felt that as children that was all we needed, but I needed them to tell me they loved me. Today I accept them for who they were, which are human beings doing the best they could based on what they knew at the time.

The biggest difference between both families is that after Papa died, I was left alone for a short period of time in the evening; however, I still felt loved, wanted, and accepted. With my secondary family, there was always someone home with me, and yet I felt unwanted and unappreciated. I take a lot of the responsibility for feeling alone—I was not willing to let them in at the time. I did what I thought was best to protect myself from feeling abandoned yet again.

Looking back, the most important thing I learned is that both families used food to show me love, when what I really needed was their attention. I discovered that when I stuffed myself with food, I could bury my feelings. With eating I didn't have to feel disappointed or deal with the loss of a loved one.

The relationships we share with family members shape our lives for what we attract, until that need within is healed by ourselves. It shows us who we are and gives us the opportunity to heal from within. Parents and caregivers set us up for life lessons; they are the stimulus, and we are then set out to uncover the message.

Then we have our siblings providing us with challenges and preparing us for the critics of the world. They always seem to know the right buttons to push to allow us to experience, learn, and grow from within. Siblings help us deal with and solve conflicts with others and within ourselves. We learn how to share and deal with power struggles.

Food

The greatest pain of my life was being frequently left alone in the evening as a child. This event left me feeling lost, isolated, abandoned, shunned, and ignored. This single event scarred me my entire life. Each time I've craved love and affection, I turn to food. In my first book, *Weight Loss for Life,* I asked the question why I was addicted to food instead of all the other things in the world. Today I know the answer: that's what I was given by all my caregivers when they couldn't be there for me. I internalized their actions as saying, "Althea, you're on your own. Now, shut up and have some cake."

I have known this for a while and am now looking at it differently so that I can finally accept it. I am ready to let go of this pain that has been feeding my excessive weight gain from 13 years old until today, the end of my 48th year. This is the seventh phase of my life, where miracles happen.

My childhood relationships with both families have taught me that I can use food for behaviour modification. I sometimes use it to beat myself up for being where I don't want to be, doing what I don't want to do, and staying with others whom I don't care to be around at that moment. I also use food as a tool to calm and comfort myself. It's a weapon to control my temper and soften my mood, and I use it to be liked and accepted. It worked well in the short-term, but long-term it's putting my life at risk with excessive weight gain, obesity, high blood sugar levels, insomnia, fits of rage, a weight-loss and weight-gain roller coaster.

The bottom line is that my challenge with food abuse is a result of me being angry at myself for being in toxic relationships with others who are sucking the life out of me. I'm afraid of being alone, so I settle for these unfulfiling relationships. I acknowledge the fact that I'm much happier when I don't talk to or see these energy vampires who always deplete my energy each time I'm in contact with them.

So, when will I stop reaching out and encouraging them to remain in my life? It about believing that I deserve to be where I want to be, doing what makes me happy with people who are fun-loving and interesting. It's a lot of work to put on a happy face when I'm burning up inside!

Knowing all this, what must I do to take of all this excess weight once and for all? I must replace the pain of being left to fend for myself with the knowledge that I did nothing wrong. I've only been living the way I was taught by those who told me they loved me. I did not know any better, so I couldn't do better—until now.

Let's look at my weight. Based on my life experiences, I do know that by eating vegetables, protein, and fruits, and by power walking three to four times each week, I will lose weight. I also know that I feel better physically, and I'm mentally alert. So why do I continue to binge on harmful foods? As mentioned earlier, it's to avoid the pain of being alone. It's also about putting myself out there where I can be seen. And there lies the truth: what if no one recognizes all my hard work? Then why do I want to lose weight? Who is it for? The last time I was at my goal weight, I was not rewarded by the universe, so I thought, *Why not gain the weight back? What's the point of doing something if I'm not going to be recognized for it? What's the point if my work is not going to be acknowledged?*

My motivation for maintaining a strong, lean, healthy body for life is feeling loved, wanted, appreciated, accepted, and acknowledged for who I am and what I've accomplished.

WEIGHT AND HOME

Belonging

There are three simple steps to balancing your home centre. The first thing to look at is your ideal city and neighbourhood to call home. In doing so, you must keep in mind where you work and decide whether you are willing to commute. If you are willing to commute, then for how long? When you are not working, what do you enjoy doing in your spare time? Are these activities available in your neighbourhood? What amenities are vital for you to call this your city? How important is it to have supermarkets, restaurants, gym, bike trails, and transit systems nearby?

For most of my life, I felt that I did not belong anywhere, and that's why I was moving from place to place: I was trying to find a place I could call home. At one point I moved three times in one year, and my mom told me she had no more room under my name for any more phone numbers. Sometimes I moved for financial reasons, and at times I felt that the next neighbourhood was going to be the one.

There was a time when I felt like Humpty Dumpy in a lot of ways. As a child, the only way I knew how to survive was for parts of me to fly away during certain events and situations. I did it so often that it became normal. By doing so, I have lost and misplaced a part of me: that part that feels open enough to connect with others in a deep and spiritual way. At this point in my life, my mission is to find and reunite us all in this present moment. Metaphorically speaking, when things become uncomfortable, I fly away like a bird.

On October 15, 1999, I took possession of my condo, the first home I'd purchased for myself and by myself. It was a beautiful home in a great neighbourhood ... and yet I was miserable. It took awhile for me to realize it was not the condo—it was me. I felt that I was in a great place but did not belong. So where *did* I belong? In most of the places I had moved to over the years, the physical structures in 90 percent of them were never the problem; it was where they were located that was the issue. They did not feel like home because they were not where I belonged—excellent buildings located in the wrong place.

Back in 2003 when I moved to Vancouver, one of my favourite things to do was visit all the different neighbourhoods. In one of the local magazines there was an ad for a book store, so the book lover in me went to check it out. It was located in the Kitsilano neighbourhood—Kits for short. I remember the first time I went to Kits; it was absolutely magical.

While walking down the streets, I felt very light, energetic, and at peace. There were no negative thoughts and no food cravings. I was happy to explore and experience all the unique nuances of the neighbourhood. At least one a week I would find myself there exploring the area and loving every second of it.

Then one day on my way home, I started to notice that each time I was leaving the area, I would get angry. Why was I so angry after experiencing such an amazing day? I was leaving the place I felt most at home to go back to a place where I felt very much disconnected in mind, body, and spirit. In leaving the quaint shops, ocean, trails, and trees, I also noticed that on my way home I would stop off and pick up a dinner that was very high in fat and sugar. This was my attempt to drown my sorrows. When we are not at peace, then we tend to think of and crave unhealthy foods instead of eating healthy meals to sustain and nourish our bodies. It's not about being bigger and better; instead, it's about being the right fit. Our soul knows what it needs; all we have to do I pay attention. I could have saved myself a lot of time, energy, and money with all the moves I made if I had tuned into myself earlier. I was being guided home, but I was not ready to listen. It took awhile for me to get to this point because of my distorted perception of what a home was. It was my thinking that I should buy a beautiful new condo instead of focusing on where I belonged and where I would feel the most free and at home.

After you find the right neighbourhood, the next step is to find the right building, whether it's a house, a condo, or an apartment. Just like the neighbourhood, it must stimulate you in a positive way. I once moved into an apartment in the middle of winter, and it faced lots of mature trees and a creek. Then came spring; these mature trees got their leaves back, and I could not see the creek. I felt that I was living in a forest and was all alone. As a result, I felt depressed because I could not see through the trees.

It's interesting because a few months after moving in, another suite in the adjacent building became available, and I jumped at the chance to move. I was talking to one of my neighbours, and she said she was feeling blue when at home; she didn't want to get up or do anything, and she did not know why until I mentioned it.

Knowing that my apartment at the time was a depressing

place to be, I avoided going home after work by trolling around and looking for food to soothe my spirit. I was going to the supermarket, buying large amounts of food, and eating it in front of the television day after day.

It does not matter if you are buying or renting. When you enter a place, look at how you are feeling when you first see it. Were you excited? What does it remind you of? What does it look like, feel like, and smell like? How does it compare to your ideal home? If you purchase it, will you be happy? Is this where you see yourself for the next 5 and 10 years, and beyond?

It's very important that you pay attention to how you are feeling in each moment. I've learned that when I'm happy, I'm exactly where I belong. When I'm feeling angry, I must look at why I'm there. What's my payoff for being there when I'm feeling so unhappy? Without the acknowledgement of your feelings, you binge to bury these feelings deep within. Examine how you feel when you are at home alone versus when you are with others. Notice how you feel as you are travelling from neighbourhood to neighbourhood, from city to city. Our food cravings are telling us where we do or do not belong.

Bad things happens to good people regardless of where you live; however, the area you choose to make your home must be a neighbourhood in which you feel comfortable walking home alone at night. It does not matter where you choose to make your home; what's important is whether you feel safe in mind, body, and spirit.

Currently I'm living in Vancouver, on the notorious Lower Eastside. I would not live remotely close to there because I do not feel safe in the day, much less at night. On the other hand, I have lots of friends who feel that it's one of the best neighbourhoods. For them they are right, and for me I'm right. Where you live and how your home is set up is based on how you are feeling about yourself. Where and how you live your life today has a very strong impact on your weight. As I've been saying all along, we turn to food for comfort because something in life is out of balance. Successful long-term weight management is about identifying what and where it is, and then doing something about it. Our weight is speaking to us—are you listening?

Looking back on my childhood, I have learned that a place is not a home. The people living inside the dwelling and how they treat each other are what constitutes a home. When my grandfather was alive, I felt that we had a home with people who loved and respected each other through their actions. After his death, the rest of us drifted apart. We still loved and respected each other, but we went off in different directions.

As a result, when my mom died, I did the same thing with my secondary family. All of a sudden I felt like an outsider. There was nothing that they did; I simply felt this way. With that experience, I set out to build my own home on my terms. There is always that one person in each family that is the glue that keeps everyone together. Once that person is gone, if someone does not step up, then everyone drifts away.

In looking back at my home in Jamaica and my teen years with my other family, I can clearly see how my upbringings have affected my home today. My Jamaican home was a beautiful, spacious home, but they were never home; everyone was always busy doing this or that. However, when we were together it was positively amazing to see all the love we had for each other.

In my second family, because I was the oldest I was expected to take care of my siblings and do most of the housework. I was forced into growing up faster than I was ready for. Then I went and bought a home in an area that was not suited for my needs. Growing up taught me that I must keep a neat, clean, and organized house, and I must buy, not rent. That caused me to be stressed and forced into buying when it was not right for me at the time. The stress came from not being prepared because I was not settled enough to buy, and as a result I stressed and binged to feel better.

I believe that I always knew where I belonged, but I was scared to take action out of fear of disappointing my family. I'm living 3000 miles away from them because this is where I belong. It's not about getting away from them; it's about me finding myself. I'm where I want to be and doing what makes me feel happy. I'm surrounded by lots of people, places, and things that bring me great joy each day. Your home is where your heart is. Are you listening to your heart?

Home Sweet Home

If you are confident in your decision as to what city and neighbourhood to call home, the next step is deciding what it looks like and then finding it. For some, where we live and with whom is the top priority in life, but for others it's not that essential. Are you living where you want to be and with the people you want?

It's been said that home is where the heart is, but what does this mean? For me, it's not about the physical building as much as it's about where I feel most comfortable. It's my own personal space where I can put my feet up, relax, and rejuvenate after a long day. I want a location where I have a great view in a fantastic neighbourhood that is close to the Pacific Ocean, with lots of walking trails. These factors far outweigh the square footage.

In fact, the best apartment I've ever had was only 500 square feet. I was brought up believing that my home should be the biggest and the best, and this cozy apartment showed me otherwise. It happened when I was looking for a one-bedroom and den in my desired neighbourhood, and I could not find any I liked. The property manager of my desired building asked me about a junior one-bedroom place. I told her I needed more space, but she said, "Take a look anyway." She had been living in one for the past several years and loved it.

The moment she opened the front door, I was sold and I told her I would take it. She responded, "Take a look first!" The reason I fell in love so quickly was that as I opened the door, the first thing I noticed was the ocean. Across from the ocean was a beautiful park. I spent many days and nights watching people walking and jogging on the seawall and playing in the park. It was also the perfect spot when there was a full moon, because the moon's image bounced off the water. Getting up early and walking the seawall was one of my favourite things to do.

After taking a closer look at the apartment, I was very happy to see that most of my things would fit. A junior one-bedroom is basically a bedroom that would fit a double bed, a side table, and nothing else, so I gave my dresser to a friend. The kitchen was a great size with lots of storage. The living room and dining room combo was a little on the small size, but it was perfect for me. I gave my dining room furniture to another friend because I never used it anyway, and then I purchased a smaller one for the kitchen. I then used the dining room area as my den; I had more than 500 books and a beautiful oak desk. I was so at peace with where I was living that there was no need to binge on unhealthy foods; instead I was involved in lots of outdoor activities that helped manage my weight.

I believe your home is your castle and should represent your personality. It's the place that you feel the safest and most comfortable. It's a place where you can be yourself in whatever way that is most comfortable for you. When we are feeling safe and comfortable, then we eat nutrient-rich foods that nourish our mind, body, and spirit.

When I was growing up in Jamaica, I always felt safe when I had my immediate family around. There was something scary about being alone that I could not explain at the time. It took many years for me to see and admit to myself that I'm scared of being alone—which is interesting because that's the way I've set up my adult life. The majority of my evenings are spent alone watching mindless television and eating massive amounts of unhealthy food. I turned toward food because I was afraid, and I attempted to suppress the fear of being alone. In a way I was reliving my childhood all over again.

So why was I choosing to live alone? On a subconscious level I felt that it was the lesser of two evils. As mentioned in the relationships chapter, I had a very unstable childhood with lots of bad examples of what marriages and families are all about. There have been numerous studies on family dynamics. As children we either run away or toward what we learn at home. At times we are not consciously aware of our behaviours. If all I'm doing is giving, and receiving very little in return, then I was choosing to be without.

The problem with that logic is we all need love and affection to thrive and grow as humans. Without the consistent giving of love, we turn to other means in an attempt to feel better. In my case I turned to food because as a child, I was taught food was love. You might feel differently, but for me a place is not a home unless I can share it with another person.

The view from that small apartment made me feel that I was part of something. I was not alone as I looked out my window and saw all the amazing people enjoying the area, and it made me want to join them. This was what was missing when I was living in another place that was twice the size; the mature trees kept me locked in. In a way the larger place felt like a closet, whereas the smaller place felt like a mansion full of loving, joyous people.

It can be fun to have time alone; in fact, I do recommend you do it often. It's not so much fun going home to an empty apartment day in and day out. It does not matter how amazing the house or apartment is; after a while we will miss having someone to share it with. As much as I love watching television, I find it's more fun watching with someone else.

Another reason I chose to be alone was because I'd not found the right people with whom to spend my time. I like people that I can give and take with, just like a tennis match. Many times I was asked what I was willing to give up to be in a relationship. I don't believe we have to give up anything; I believe a relationship is a partnership designed to enhance what we already have. If we give up the things we love for the sake of a relationship, then after a while we will end up resenting or even hating the other person.

Instead of giving up things, I believe in being honest and up front with the other person as to what's important to each of us. What can we live with and without? Our home must be a reflection of who we both are. It's not my house or your house—it's our home.

Regardless of how amazing our professional life is, we need to come back to our home base to rest and rejuvenate. It must be a comfortable place where you can be yourself, free of makeup and pretence. You must be surrounded by only the best and the most comfortable people and things. Not the biggest—only the best will so. For me size does not matter; I prefer quality instead of the quantity. If you are not comfortable living where you are, then it's time to consider the pros and cons of moving versus staying put.

Moving is not always about moving. Sometimes it's about the natural progression of life. Despite having free will, we can't rush the process. To move from one stage to the next, we must first complete the assignment from before. We must first learn the lesson because it sets up the next stage. Moving on before the lesson is learned is like moving to another country and not speaking the language. The natives are speaking, yet you don't understand what they are saying. Before you can make a place your home, you must first understand what it is you really want and need in a home. What is your definition of a home?

If your house or apartment does not feel like a home, then moving may or may not be the answer. You can make anywhere your home if you are feeling at home with and within yourself. Take a good look at what's really missing in the home, neighbourhood, city, and even country in which you currently reside.

Our childhood home is full of memories, and that's extremely powerful. It's so impactful that I use it as a measuring stick in my adulthood. All the numerous moves I made in my 20s and 30s were about attempting to find what I'd lost after Papa died: the closeness, the jokes, the laughter, and the connection I felt living with him and the rest of the family in my childhood home. As much as I care about my new family, I was not able to recreate the feelings from my original family.

It makes sense that I was not able to duplicate the feelings of being safe and secure, because they are different people here to give and teach me new experiences. The problem was that I was not ready to see or accept this lesson no matter how loving they were. I was still living in the past, and when people are living in the past, then there is no room for anyone else. It's as if I was stuck in a holding pattern for many years. To receive love, we must be open to receive love. No one can take Papa's place in my heart, and therefore there is no reason to fear him being replaced.

If it does not feel right, then it's something you must change to bring about happiness. Moving is not a bad thing, providing you are consciously aware of why you are moving.

So here you are in your ideal city, neighbourhood, and home, and yet you are having difficulty maintaining your strong, lean, and healthy weight. Why? It's now time to look at what activities you are involved in that lead you to binge. You did your homework and are blessed with everything you have asked for, so why are you being so self-destructive?

For me, the biggest home activity is too much time home alone watching television. I'm 3000 miles away from my family, and when I don't want to talk to anyone, in that moment I turn to food for comfort. I watch something I don't want to because I am bored, and it leads to binge eating for me.

The two emotions that drive us are love and fear. Love motivates us to go out and explore what the world has to offer: meeting new people and engaging in new activities. On the other hand, fear will keep us stuck in our home, eating ourselves sick and sometimes into an early grave. In this case, the fear of being consumed by the needy people in our lives and the fear of going out and meeting new people results in being bored.

You know what you must do, but you are afraid to do it. What if you put yourself out there, and you are then rejected for being yourself? What if you put yourself out there, and you find yourself around the same personalities from which you have been trying to get away? It's the same people but different times, places, and faces, with the same results.

I don't know about you, but I tend to eat more when I'm home alone. For years I could not understand it because I absolutely love my home. It was not the home; it was being alone, the not having anyone with whom to share my life. The obsessive food thoughts were telling me to call on family and friends, and I was resisting. I needed to share myself with others, and for some reason I did not want to. In order to shut out the message, I turned to food to cover up and suppress my true nature as a social butterfly. I was afraid of getting hurt, so I chose not to let others get close to me.

I do have a choice because I have free will. I can choose not to move into the direction I am being led and be miserable, or I can choose to accept this challenge of moving into a new direction and see what happens. I can choose to stay stuck doing the same old thing, or I can choose to take another path despite not knowing where this gravel road may lead.

As I was writing the above, I realized that the only time I don't feel the need to eat is when I am writing. Writing takes away the aloneness I feel when I'm home alone. As a child I would get lost in reading, and today I get lost in putting my feelings down on paper. With that said, it does not mean that I'm barricading myself in my ivory tower, locked away from the rest of the world. Yes, I do need time by myself; however, it's a Healthea choice to share my home, thoughts, feelings, and myself with others. My home is to be shared, and I choose to share it with loved ones.

"Be open to everything and attached to nothing." To me, this means walking through all open doors. It means accepting people, places, and things for who and what they are, and accepting the lessons they are here to teach me. It's not necessary to be afraid of letting new things into my life because at some point one of us will be leaving. Without the interaction with others, we are unable to learn certain lessons. Everything that happens in life is for a reason, no matter how challenging it might seem in the moment. I ask, "What lesson am I to learn from this event, person, or place?" All events are an opportunity to learn something about us. With that said, what lesson was in the aloneness I feel when home alone?

Althea, just give thanks for what you have today. I have a beautiful life and home to be shared with others. Thank you for being a participant in my life and teaching what I must learn. I must stay put and accept what it is that I have, the gifts that I am being offered in this moment. To see, I must open my eyes; to hear, I must open my ears; to know, I must open my heart; to feel, I must open my mind and accept what is.

Earlier this year I asked myself, "How can someone who has so much be so unhappy?" The answer is because I'm not being myself. I am approaching life according to what I believe society wants.

Once I found my home in Vancouver, it was time to stop moving and focus on my career path. I felt stuck in a dead-end profession for years because I did not feel at home. Then came these food cravings, which I gave into instead of focusing on what I was really feeling in that particular moment. My past homes did not lead me to binge; instead it was my fear of facing my own feelings and of not knowing where I belong. Once I started to pay attention, I soon realized that all I had to do was admit to myself that I crave food in the evenings as a lack of love and affection for where I was living.

Today my home is a peaceful place where I relax, sleep, and rejuvenate. Home is a peaceful place for exercise and rest. Lack of sleep increases cortisol, which increase belly fat. I binge on unhealthy foods when home alone because I'm afraid of being alone.

What have I learned from the past that's positive? Well, over the years living alone has taught me that I need others in order to grow and survive. Constant thoughts of what to eat when I'm home alone mean that my soul is crying out to be fed and nurtured by the love of another. It's my heart telling me to stop and look at what I'm doing, feeling, and thinking. I've learned that to be truly happy in my home life, I must let go of traditions that were not working and embrace the ones that are. It's okay for me to change and try new things that make me happy. A building is not a home; it's the people inside the building that makes it a home. Buying a house or condo is not a home. A home is what you make of it. You can make a home out of anything. What I loved most about living with my second family was weekends and holidays, the times we spent eating and talking around the dining room table. I usually laughed far more than I ate.

How have these experiences made me the person I am today? To manage my weight without dieting, I put down roots in one place. I do travel, but I have a home base to which I can come back. With stability comes fewer food cravings, and with fewer cravings comes a clear mind, a healthy body, and a happy spirit.

To have what you truly want need and desire, you must first know what you are looking for. Below are a few questions to get you started. As before, please take a few minutes in a quiet place and think about your answers. It's not about what your family and friends want—it's all about what *you* need to feel comfortable, happy, and content in your home. Reexamine your answers at least two more times over a period of a week to make sure it's really what you need.

If you are married, it's a good idea for both of you to complete this activity individually and then come together and compare notes. Then compile a composite, ensuring both of you are happy with the list. Something to consider is having a section for each, such as a man cave for him and an activity or craft area for her. There is no right or wrong way, just what's best for you both.

- What do you require? You must know where you want to be, with whom, and how to use this space.
- How many rooms, and what are each used for?
- What is too big or too small?
- What's the purpose of this place? What will it be used for—home, business, or a combination?

With all the moves I have made over the years trying to find the right home, I realized that just like Dorothy in *The Wizard of Oz,* home is within me. It's feeling at home with and within myself. Yes, living in the right neighbourhood is necessary, because living in the right area helps you become at peace, and when you are at peace you are more relaxed and are less likely to binge eat. I've also learned that a home is to be shared. You will have the perfect home in your ideal neighbourhood when you get real with yourself by answering the tough questions that you have been afraid to ask.

Organized Space

Part of balancing your home centre is ensuring it's clean, neat, and organized at all times. A clean home means a clear mind and making space for others to join me. Having a schedule helps. Some people do not like cleaning, but you have to make a choice to have someone come in and do it or else schedule it into your week. I find that by doing a little bit each day and cleaning up after myself, it does not take a lot of time. Often all I have to do is vacuum and dust once weekly; the rest I do a little each day.

When things pile up, then it takes much more time and effort to complete tasks. Here are a few examples of what I do on a daily basis. These things take only a few minutes each day but save me a ton of time later.

- Wipe down stove and sinks after each use.
- After undressing, hang up clothes or place them in hamper for washing.
- Wash dishes after each meal.
- Never go to bed with dirty dishes in the sink.
- Have enough essentials, such as underwear and towels, so that I only have to do laundry once a month.
- Hire a cleaning lady or trade with a friend for other services (babysitting, carpooling).
- Dust, mop, and vacuum when I have the most energy. For me, it's at midnight or first thing in the morning, after I wake up.

WEIGHT AND GROWTH

Personal Growth and Development

There are lots of experts out there who differ in their definitions of personal growth and development. For me, they are being open to learning, growing, and advancing your belief system to meet your immediate needs and desires. It's about being receptive to new ideas and new ways of thinking, being, and living. It's expanding and advancing your physical, emotional, intellectual, spiritual, and social awareness to improve and inspire yourself to reach your full potential. It's expanding your self-awareness and self-knowledge of who you are, what you are, and what you do. It's being comfortable in your own skin.

I am often asked, "How do personal growth and development affect weight?" Being overweight is a clear indication that something in your life is out of balance. We eat large amounts of unhealthy foods to cover up and suppress our displeasure of what we are experiencing. Often we turn to food because we are afraid or uncomfortable to see things the way they are. To acknowledge something is wrong means that we have to fix it. At times we may feel it's easier to deny our feelings, but in the long run that's detrimental to our health and well-being.

When we focus on weight loss, then we are treating the symptom but not the cause. That's why after we lose the weight, we quickly put it back on as a result of not addressing the cause of our weight gain. When we address the cause, then we can make a conscious decision to change this destructive behaviour and replace it with a Healthea way of living.

As I've mentioned before, despite the dangerous effects of most diets, they do help one losing weight. On the other hand, to maintain this weight loss along with eating healthy and regular exercise, we must identify and treat the imbalance in our lives. Personal growth and development means to develop certain coping skills to identify and elevate our personal triggers before they are blown out of proportion. We must face the music to understand their messages.

It took me several decades to understand that the reason I was overweight was a direct result of my being in the wrong career. As a store manager I was very successful, but I've always known that I do not belong there. This was abundantly clear to me a few years ago, when the company I was working for took the entire store manager team of more than 3000 people to Las Vegas. Here we were at the MGM Grand Hotel, and everyone was laughing and having a good time. At one point I mentally pulled away from the group and simply watched. They were all genuinely have a great time, and I was faking being interested in conversation. It was at that point I said to myself, *I don't belong here!*

Many years later, I realized my life's work was to help women on a deeper level. Each time I helped an unhappy woman buy a new outfit, I knew deep down that it was just a temporary fix. To solve her body and self-esteem issues, I needed to find out what was going on in her life. I needed to know whether she was happy with her career, finances, home, relationships, spirituality, health and fitness, and personal growth and development.

When our person growth and development life centre is out of balance, it's because we are stuck in a rut. We are doing the same things day in and day out with the same people. We are not trying new things such as reading books, attending seminars, or even taking a different route home from work. We are afraid to go deep within and explore. We are afraid to embrace the essence of who we really are.

Every day millions of people lose weight only to regain it. For several seasons *The Biggest Loser* was one of my favourite TV shows. The winner of season three, Eric Chopin, lost more than half his body weight. At 36 years old he went from 407 pounds to 193 pounds to become the biggest loser. He then regained 122 of those pounds because he did not address the underlining reasons for his weight gain in the first place.

He won the show and the prize money of $250,000. Then the studio lights dimmed and the promotional tours ended. Now he found himself in the same place he was mentally and emotionally before he went on the show. He was asking the same question that millions of us continue to ask ourselves until we accept our truth: "I'm at my goal weight—now what?"

On the other hand, look at Ali Vincent, who was the season five winner and made a career out of it because she'd found the answer to her question, "Now what?" She is the author of *Believe It, Be It: How the Biggest Loser Won Me Back My Life*. Ali is also a spokesperson for 24 Hour Fitness. She proves my point that to successfully manage weight loss, we must first address the root cause of *why* we put on the weight in the first place.

After publishing *Weight Loss for Life,* I did not ask the question, "Now what?" And I ended up regaining most of the weight. As a result I was even more determined to understand why I would put myself in this position yet again. I started out by exploring this question: "Why am I resisting keeping off this 45 extra pounds I'm carrying around?" Then I realized it was about routine.

For me, routine is boring as hell, yet it gets the job done. After we lose the weight, most of us abandon the routine that got us our desired results. Practice is doing something over and over again until it becomes habit. Anyone who has lost weight has proved that we do know how to commit to achieving a certain goal. It takes practice, dedication, and commitment to be successful in losing the weight in the first place. We must do the same thing when we are at the maintenance stage. It's a lifestyle change, not a diet, and it must be treated accordingly. I know that for me to lose weight, all I have to do is get up early four times a week and go on a power walk for more than two hours. I have a protein shake for breakfast and fruit for a mid-morning snack. Then I have protein and vegetables for lunch; nuts, seeds, or raw vegetables for an afternoon snack; and dinner.

Before we reach our weight goals, we must start planning the weight management stage. If you wait until you are at your goal weight, then it's too late because it opens up the door for old habits to resurface. For example, I know that for my physical health, I must continue power walking, so I map out different routes to keep it fresh. I also took up hiking to keep it interesting. I then determine how I'm going to integrate grain products into my diet twice per week. Writing is an activity that fuels my soul, so I get up at 6:00 a.m. to write before I go to work. On my day off, I'm at the library writing before 11:00 a.m.

Here is my complete list for maintaining my weight. Thus

far on my journey as a spiritual being who is here to have a human experience, this is what I know works for me to balance my life centres and maintain my desired weight.

- Health and Fitness—Do physical exercise.
- Spirituality—Meditate.
- Career—Do what I love, feel passionate about, and have fun doing.
- Finances—Do something each day to bring balance to my life.
- Home—Live where I have peace of mind.
- Relationships—Embrace all people, places, and things that nurture me.
- Personal Growth and Development—Study, write, and teach weight management.

As a weight management specialist, my focus is placed on where you want to be in life and how you will get there. In *The Giant Within,* Tony Robins says that to get what we want, me must, "Focus on what you want instead of what you don't want because you already have what you don't want." We are already overweight, so why are we focusing on weight?

How many times have you told yourself that you need to lose weight … and then you do nothing about it? What's stopping you from following through? Why do you cheat on your diet? What's stopping you from being successful? Is it fear, and if so, of what? What are you doing today to sabotage yourself? What's the point of stressing out over your weight if you have no intention of losing the weight?

I'm asking these questions because for years I've been trying to lose weight by focusing on weight loss. I'm here to tell you that the best way to lose weight—and keep it off permanently—is to frequently eat healthy food, exercise daily, and live a balanced life. Expend more energy than you take in. For me, focusing on weight loss increased my stress level, resulting in binge eating and excessive weight gain. On the other hand, focusing on what I need in the here and now to get to my goal does the trick. The weight is simply the symptom, not the root.

Instead of focusing on what to eat, I find what works best for me is to focus on where I want to be. Where do I see myself? Based on past experiences, I narrowed it down to the following list: what I love, feel passionate about, and have fun doing in this moment. By concentrating on these areas, I decreased my stress levels and my appetite for binge eating when not hungry. I've discovered that I turn to food when I'm where I don't want to be.

Conflict for Growth

Everyone who enters your life will have an impact, whether it's positive or negative. All interactions are designed to show us who we are, what we are, and how we have been acting. There is no such thing as an accidental meeting; the next several pages will demonstrate this point.

During my quest for living a strong, lean, healthy, and balanced life, I realized that insights into the person we are can come from anywhere, including our family, friends, a movie, a television show, or even a complete stranger. This chapter is about one of the most painful periods along my path, and yet it's one of the most fulfiling times for me. This was a time where I was forced to look deep within myself and question the motives of everyone around me, including myself. I was forced to go deeper within myself in order to uncover the truth of who I am and my true purpose that I have been subconsciously suppressing.

For years I was working in a profession that no longer served me, so I decided to go back to school. I came into contact with the Private College after picking up their brochure at a health show. After reading it I realized that it contained all the elements that I was looking for in a career. I knew that I wanted to help others by bringing clarity and understanding to their lives through coaching and counselling, because of my own challenge with my weight and the need to help others with their emotional issues. I knew that I overeat due to my emotional hang-ups, and I wanted to learn how to deal with the issues at hand instead of turning to food. I believed that once I solved my own mystery, I would be able to turn it into a career for helping others.

After meeting with the vice president of the college, I chose to enrol in the Wellness Diploma Program. It was 57 weeks consisting of three months of counselling, three months of coaching life skills, and six months of wellness, plus a four-week practicum that would result in a diploma at the end. I chose Private College because it promised to teach me how to us the proper tools necessary to solve emotional issues that prevented individuals from moving forward in life. I was extremely excited about starting school and being trained in a new and rewarding career.

Upon starting college, my intention was to figure out my place in the world. I needed a place for gathering information on what to do next with my life in order to feel fulfiled as a human and a spiritual being. I was looking for confirmation and understanding in several areas. I needed to understand why I was running away from romantic relationships with a man who was fun-loving and who shared my interests—someone who loved me and wouldn't try to change me. I told myself that it was what I wanted, and yet I did all that I could to keep him at bay. Another goal was finding financial stability so that I could live my life of purpose, which was to study, write, and teach weight management to obese women.

The Private College's philosophy is experiential learning, meaning that we are expected to bring our experiences, issues, and challenges as part of our training on how to effectively coach and counsel our clients. Over the years I have uncovered a lot about myself, but I wanted to discover the essence of Althea. What is the one thing that oozes out of my pores, that is my gift to the world? It was about narrowing down my choices so that I could be more specialized and effective. This is the thing that I am to give to the world freely and without attachment. Finally I wanted to know how to be one with the universe. I was looking to increase my spiritual connection so that I could understand my clients and myself more completely. After that the goal was to put those conclusions into an action plan for starting my new career. In the meantime I would sharpen my communication skills and interact with like-minded people at college.

It did not turn out the way I thought it would. Instead what I found was a situation where I felt very much alone and isolated. Once again I found myself in a place where I didn't want to be. I was with a group of people who did not care about who I was as an individual; for them, it was about lumping everyone into the same category.

The select few who I considered to be bullies felt that I appeared too happy and well-adjusted, and therefore I must be hiding some deep-rooted, traumatic events from my past—and they were determined to get it out of me. All they cared about knowing was my so-called secrets. These secrets didn't exist. They felt that because they had secrets, I must have them as well, and by uncovering my secret pains they would be able to fix me. In a way I can understand where they were coming from, because most of them were recovering drug addicts, alcoholics, prostitutes, and convicts. Their childhoods were very traumatic; most had been molested, raped, and physically and mentally abused. Some had great families and support systems, but others did not.

They could not understand that I'd had a great childhood for the most part. I shared my feelings surrounding my conception, being raised by my maternal grandparents from 3 months old, and the fact that I was physically abused a couple of times by one uncle, but I have forgiven him.

They thought it wasn't possible to move on and that there was more to it. They actually told me that there was more to me that what I said, even though I made it clear that I was not perfect and had simply done a lot of work on myself over the years. A select few of my classmates felt that my challenges and experiences were not traumatic enough to be used as a stimulus for the group—that I was cheating the group by not opening up more.

I believe that when others are eager to hear the negative aspects of your life, it's because they are extremely uncomfortable with people who are happy. They are unsure of how to deal with or handle the positive people or situations because they are used to negativity. They find it difficult to believe that others have done the hard work by facing their past, forgiving people, and being happy and content with their pasts.

As I mentioned earlier, there are three parts to the full program; however, students also had the option of only taking the coaching class for a life skills certificate, or they could take the coaching and counselling programs for a life coach and life skills instructor diploma. Depending on when you start, you can be in a class with others from all three groups. For example, when I started it was in the counselling program, where there were 19 students, six of whom were finishing up the full Wellness Diploma Program, two were finishing up the Life Skills Diploma Program, and the remaining 11 us were new students.

The first day we were told that we would be divided into groups of threes and called a triad. All we were told was that our triad met each morning at 9:00 a.m.; we were also told that there would be at least one member from the graduating class to help us if we had any questions about how things worked. In my triad, Mary was from the graduating class, and Wayne was a newcomer like I was.

The second day in triad, Mary asked me how I was feeling, and I said fine. She then questioned me at length because in her opinion, being fine was not a feeling. I did not understand where she was going with her response to me, or why my answer was not good enough. I then got very defensive because I felt attacked. This was a person whom I'd known for all of 24 hours, and she was now telling me how I should feel. In the end I felt that I was not being heard or understood, and therefore my opinions, thoughts, and ideas were not valued. I believe that I reacted this way because she was treating me the way all my previous employers had treated me, feeding into my insecurities that without understanding there is lack of intelligence. She made me feel that I was stupid and didn't know what I was doing, which put me on a mission to show others how smart I was.

In the past I would have withdrawn myself from the group if I felt that I was not being listened to or acknowledged. I was feeling left out, like I didn't have anything in common with my triad. I recognized on my own that this was not a good way of dealing with conflicts, and so the following day I told Mary how I felt about the previous day's interaction. She also shared her feelings, and in the end we decided that we must listen more and ask questions to verify the other's intention before jumping to conclusions and hurting each other's feelings. We both felt very good about our talk afterward.

I learned from this exchange that it's okay not to understand, because it's not a sign of weakness; rather, it's an opportunity to learn and grow as a person. It's time to stop obsessing and pay attention to what others are saying without judging them. I then came to the conclusion that I was choosing not to understand, because if I understood then I would have to change, and I was afraid of changing due to my insecurities about my ability to do well in my new profession, where I didn't have any formal experience. It also taught me that when others irritate me, it's because they are mimicking my behaviour; they are showing me how I am treating myself at that time. When I am treating myself well, then the behaviours of others are irrelevant to me, and they can't push my buttons.

Looking back on the first week, Monday was a so-so day, and Tuesday and Wednesday were getting worse because I did not understand most of what Jennifer, the instructor, was saying. It all started on Tuesday morning when I sat in the seat I was in the previous day. Jennifer then asked who was sitting in the same seat as the previous day, and I raised my hand along with a few more people. She went on to imply that it was a sign of rigidity for consistently sitting in the same seat.

I then had a five-minute discussion with her explaining that I was in the same seat because I perceived it to be the most comfortable seat, and I must be comfortable if I was to be here for seven hours. I told her that I would be comfortable moving to another seat in the room, but I was more comfortable by the window. She left it at that, and of course I changed seats daily to show her that I was flexible. From the exchanges between Kimberley and Jennifer, I learned that my need to explain myself to others is my attempt to convince myself that I am okay, that I am smart, and that I do know what I am doing and talking about.

The week continued downhill from there, and everything came to a head on Thursday. During morning class, I was feeling very tired and uninterested in what Jennifer was saying, and I found it hard to stay awake. The way the days were set up, after triad we had an hour and a half of what was called clearings. That's when we put issues that we had with our classmates on the table, where they could be discussed and then solved. For example, one classmate—let's call her May— cleared with classmate June because May believed that June was breaking one of the class rules by having an affair with classmate Paul, and both parties denied it. An argument then went on for 40 minutes between them. May had absolutely no proof of the affair; she then admitted to other classmates that she was jealous of the friendship between June and Paul.

I thought, *Who cares who is sleeping with whom? It's only affecting the class because May decided to stick her nose into their business. If May would just mind her own business by concentrating on her own dysfunctional life, then all will be well.* Until she had proof that they were lovers instead of best friends, as they had been saying, I didn't want to hear what May had to say on the matter. Accusation without proof only causes suspicion and mistrust among classmates.

I felt that 90 percent of clearings were a waste of time because the instructor encouraged us to create situations with each other so that we could solve them. Clearings were initiated when a classmate had an issue with another on any and all issues, including someone wearing too much makeup, dressing too formally for class, not talking enough in class, talking too much in class, not sharing enough past hurt, sharing too much past history, crying too much, being a phony, having a poor attendance record, being too well-adjusted, or being part of a clique.

At times I would be so disgusted with what took place during clearings that I wanted to take off at lunchtime. On one such occasion I was so upset that I took my lunch with me and went for a walk by myself, to get away from all the negativity of the morning. When I arrived at school, I was usually in a happy and upbeat mood. After clearings I was usually down in the dumps because of all the negative energy in the classroom, even if I was not directly involved.

As I was talking down Broadway, I asked myself what was wrong. Why was I feeling sad? I was finally in the program I desperately wanted to get into and had been looking forward to it for months, but it was not working for me. In fact, all this program had shown me thus far was how cruel we could be to each other. I finally said to myself that all I wanted was to find my place in the world. Why was it so difficult to do?

I then saw a man who appeared to be homeless sitting on the sidewalk, so I proceeded to look for change in my wallet. I then noticed that he did not have a hat, cup, or any kind of container for the change, so I decided not to offer him the money because he was not asking me for it. I put the money back into my wallet and continued walking. When I got to the Book Warehouse, I stopped to look at the titles in the first window. There was nothing of interest, so I went over to their second window.

A girl holding up a UNICEF sign asked if she could have a word with me, and after hesitating I agreed. She went on to tell me how the organization helped people from all over the world, but after a few minutes I realized that tears were welling up within me. I then asked her for a card because I couldn't listen at this time. She told me that she did not have a card but that I could find more information at unicef.com. She saw that I was upset and said that she was sorry. I told her that it was not her; I had simply been having a bad day.

I then went off down the street crying, so I decided to find a quiet place. I ended up in a parking lot in a secluded area and burst out crying for about 10 minutes while thinking that I was suppressing my natural instincts. I then headed back to school, but I then started to think about how for years I had been suppressing my natural instincts, and again the waterworks started to flow. I saw steps leading to a parking lot and decided to sit down and let it all out. I cried for another 10 minutes, which made me feel much better. I then went back to school.

When I got home, my friend Iris called, and I told her what had happened. She then told me that it was probably because I'd invested a lot of myself both financially and emotionally into this program, and I was very disappointed because it was not what I'd thought it was going to be. My friend Laurie from Toronto called and said the same thing.

I then told Laurie about having to give a presentation, and she responded with the question, "What is it about?" I told her how I overcame my fear of speaking in public. She then replied, "Is that the worst thing you had to overcome in life?" My response was yes. Laurie then asked, "What about the death of your mother?" I told her that I didn't have enough to talk on the subject for a minimum of 10 minutes. Laurie then told me that I could speak about how my life was changing and how it got me where I was today. I then told her that I didn't want to share all that with these people.

After I got off the phone, I started to think about my

conversation with Laurie. I was getting more and more upset with each thought of having to share something so personal with a group of strangers who were so different from me. At the same time, I did not want to face the fact that if I opened up to them, then this would bring me closer to them. I then asked the question, "Who I am doing this for—them or me?" I realized that I was acting like a spoiled brat. I then started to think of what I would say if I decided to take Laurie's advice, and I started to cry uncontrollably because I realized how much I missed Mom.

The following day during clearing session and before the presentation, I told the group about my meltdown over the previous day and my indecision about which presentation to do. The group said that they appreciated my telling them and that they now felt closer to me. This left me fuming on the inside because I believed that the class loved those who were in pain and tried to rip others apart if they appeared to be strong and well-adjusted. The select few who were encouraged by the instructor were not happy unless everyone else was unhappy as well.

There was a situation where Joan, a classmate, called out Annette and two other classmates for being hypocrites. She felt that they were not being genuine in their feelings and were ganging up on another student for something that everyone else did. After 10 minutes (which seemed like a lifetime) of both going back and forth with insults, Joan then finally had enough, and she called Annette a few bad words and left the class, slamming the door behind her.

This was a regular occurrence between the bullies and the rest of the class, so I was not surprised. What was shocking was that after Joan left the room, Annette pumped her fist in the air and said, "Yes! That needed to come out of her." And the instructor agreed. That was when I realized that the goal of some students was to get others so angry that they would have a problem to fix. They were creating a problem where one did not exist in order to practice their coaching and counselling skills.

I have been telling myself that I want to be heard; however, I put myself in positions and situations where it's almost impossible for me to be heard. I do this by sitting in the back of classrooms, not participating in class readings, and trying to blend into the background. I consistently put myself in situations where I am attacked for my viewpoint and then am effectively muzzled and choose not to speak my truth. I put myself in situations where I am expected to put on my face and get in a position that is not interesting to me or that is not within my best interests, leaving me to play a part in my life instead of living purposely. I have this great power within myself; however, I consistently put myself in positions where I have to contain and suppress my power and myself. This leads me to overeat in order to suppress my rage.

This cycle is directly linked to my primary family dynamic, where I was consistently told that I was special and loved, and that everything was going to be okay. I was the centre of their world, and they took care of me. All my needs and wants were anticipated. I then moved into my secondary family with the same expectations, and when that was not reciprocated, I was left feeling lost, alone, rejected, and abandoned. It's fair to say that I put myself in groups and situations trying to duplicate the safety and security that I had and felt for the first 12 years of my life growing up in Jamaica.

To date I have been waiting for someone to come and take care of me; however, I have come to realize that he is not coming, so I must take responsibility for myself by paying my bills on time, eating correctly, exercising, and nurturing myself with love, acceptance, and integrity.

It's my opinion that if you are facing the perception that you were emotionally abandoned as a child, you may consider asking yourself how you came to this conclusion. There have been numerous times I felt this way—until one day I decided to challenge this belief, and then I realized several things. First, I was loved as a child, and I still ended up feeling unloved as an adult. Second, I was raised in a safe and secure environment, and I still ended up feeling unsafe and insecure in my environment and in my own skin. I came to the conclusion that I can blame all my challenges in life on my childhood, or I can take responsibility for my life. I figure it's time to throw caution to the wind and have some fun. That's why I fought so hard to stay focused on the here on now instead of getting pulled into the drama of the class.

People are always looking to me to lead, and I have been resisting. Why am I resisting leadership and responsibility? For me, it was a way of keeping myself from being hurt by others. I now know that I need to be around others to keep my energy moving; without them, I might feel stuck and unable to move forward or to see and think clearly.

The two types of people that I attract are those who keep me happy, and those who act as a stimulus to show me where I am stuck. I love and welcome both groups of people regardless of what package they show up in. My purpose in life is to connect with others and the universe in a meaningful way, in order to feed my soul and bring me all the joy, happiness, and fulfilment I crave.

I must do this as the teacher, not the student. It's now time to share what I have learned over the years. I now know that I am not the message; rather, I am the vessel delivering the message.

If the message is rejected, it means that the person is not ready, willing, or able to receive it at this time.

I did this because I was afraid of moving forward and of being rejected. Rejection for me is all about not being listened to or taken seriously, being dismissed like yesterday's garbage, and saying I'm not important. I was afraid of being rejected for my thoughts and ideas in my chosen profession, so I went back to school to hide, and what I got in return was the fact that I was rejected by some of my classmates for my thoughts and ideas in school. If I am going to be rejected anyway, I might as well be rejected for something that I love.

The essence of Althea is, "I choose to live in the here and now while facing head-on any and all past hurt that needs to surface, in order to release it and grow as a spiritual being."

Energy Zappers

One morning during clearing, I wanted to respond to what was being said. I knew from previous experience that putting my hand up would not help me because I would be ignored. Waiting for an opening did not seem to work because someone else always jumped in before I did. I said wanted to add something, but Steve, the counsellor of the day, said, "Sorry, Althea, Michael is first."

After Michael said what he wanted to say, Jennifer announced that clearing was now over for the day. Patricia then started to cry because she'd had her hand up and was passed over, and everyone's focus was now on her. Clearing was extended so that she got to say what she needed to say. I asked myself why I did not insist that my opinion be heard. I realized that this event showed me how I interacted with my family, which was allowing them to ignore me.

Patricia reminds me of a family member who uses his tone of voice and tears to get what he wants. I wondered what all this was trying to tell me. I love this person, and I like Patricia a lot; however, their actions disturb me deeply. I feel like they were sent to suck the life out of me, and I was not clear what to do about it.

I am wondering if it's a lesson of letting me know that I am a strong person and don't need as much attention as others. Or perhaps it's that I must be tolerant and accepting of others by listening to and valuing their opinions. Or I must instead look inside myself for what I need. Or I need to have confidence in my abilities and myself, because I know what I need and how to give it to myself. It's possible that the universe might be telling me that I will not find validation from outside myself. The other possibility is the one that I believe to be true for myself, which is that I must stand up for myself. It doesn't matter how minor I think my opinion is, I must state it. I must stand up and be counted in my life. It's about owning my voice, truth, and authentic self.

Through the following activities, I find that I am more confident in speaking my truth and getting the validation of self that I need from others and myself. I journal daily, take nature walks, and ask for what I need, and these activities eliminate the feeling of guilt about taking time for myself. I don't shut down but rather remain open to receiving. I start validating myself instead of looking for validation from people who are not capable of validating me because they are emotionally unavailable for me. In the end I realized that I am always looking for confirmation of what I know from others. This event was telling me to trust within myself that I know what's best for me. It's also for me to ask, "Am I sharing my opinion to help another person, or to feed my own ego?"

I find that people who are energy zappers are the ones who are just talking to get attention. Whining in order to make others feel sorry for them can be a trigger for us because they are showing us that we are wearing our wounds on our sleeves. Wearing wounds on the sleeve can do two things. First you will attract people who are very negative; they are the ones who are wearing their wounds on their sleeves. These people might be mirroring our own wounds, such as being overweight, having financial issues, and having challenges in love. This is to demonstrate how we have been thinking and acting in the world. Most of us are unable to see our pain until someone points it out for us.

The second thing is that the people that you really want in life will be repelled or frightened away by the pain that they can sense. These people are the ones who have shared interests and that love to have fun. They are the ones whom you truly want in your life to help you get out of your shell and into the world.

Another name for energy zappers are energy vampires. There are two types of energy vampires: the first are those who are afraid of powerful people, so they display their intentions by being very negative and consistently telling others what's wrong with them and how they should change. Their own energy is low, so by being negative they can take the other person's energy in order to feel good themselves. They are saying, "I want some of your power." All you have to do is say, "No, I don't share my power," by simply telling them, "I understand what you are saying," and then walking away from them. Sometimes they will try and zap your energy by getting you angry.

Energy vampires are great teachers because they taught me how to be with others when they are deep within their feelings. There is nothing to be afraid of because I can't be consumed by their emotions if I don't want to be. In the past, I believed that if I was consumed, then I would not be effective with them. I now know that I have nothing to worry about, because I have the ability to be empathetic during the challenging times, as well as be happy for them during their triumphant times.

Teachers in Disguise

There are key people at the Private College who have been my biggest teachers, both through their positive and negative interactions with me. These are the lessons that each person taught me.

Mary showed me that I must be mindful not to mandate how others should act or feel. Rather, I must listen carefully to my clients and ask for clarification if I'm unsure of what they mean or need in order to feel heard, accepted, and comfortable.

Jennifer taught me that I must encourage others to tell their stories their own way. I must always ask for what I want and speak my truth; this is the only way I will truly get what I want. If others don't know what I want, how can they give it to me? She taught me that I must choose my words carefully, because I am prone to using them as weapons. Learning the language of others will allow me to help more effectively.

I also realized that Jennifer reminds me of Mom and the day I told her I hated her. That was the day I learned that I could protect myself from others by using my words as a weapon. I was not aware for all those years that I was using my gift of speech to harm others. It became apparent to me that I have been avoiding nurturing others and being nurtured because of my fears of being rejected by them. "If I don't let them in, then they can't hurt me" is not protection—rather it's hiding from the world and is proven to be more painful.

Carol's lesson was how to be mindful not to impose my will and values on others. Annette showed me that I back away from strong-willed people due to my irrational fear of being consumed by others, so I tell them what they want to hear even though it's not my belief. I am a very private person because I don't like being exposed for all to see. Experts are not supposed to be vulnerable, and I don't respect vulnerability in my mentor.

Peter was my favourite teacher who showed me that I am not alone in the world, that I am normal and there is nothing wrong with me. I am not alone in thoughts and experiences; even though we are polar opposites in appearance, we are truly the same. Observing him showed me the possibilities in life. We both have a fear of being sent away if we are bad, of public speaking, and even of practical jokes.

I don't speak up because I think others will think that I am weird or crazy. Angie was only in class for two weeks, but she left a lasting impression on me by showing me how I appear in the world—how others view my appearance, posture, and actions.

Patricia reminds me not to back away from people who are consumed by emotional pain, and I am stuck in victim mode due to my irrational fear of being consumed by others. I should be mindful of my storytelling when I am with a client, because it can take the attention off the client and put it on to me, leaving them feeling sorry for me and thinking that they need to take care of me. They might think that I am trying to compete by comparing wounds, which they may view as minimizing them and their feelings.

An unusual situation happened between Patricia and me one afternoon that led me to believe that teachers show up at different times and places, and under different situations. It was August 4, 2004. After lunch I asked Patricia to join me outside for a walk. While walking up Quebec Street, she pointed out a garden in someone's backyard. I then told her that it reminded me of my parents' garden, and she said that's why she pointed it out to me. The garden had peas, some of which were overripe and needed to be picked; some were still green. There were other vegetables such as green peppers. It was a beautiful garden.

We continued to walk and talk about feeling abandoned, and I listed the circumstances in the past where I'd felt abandoned. Patricia then asked me how I felt when Carolyn, a friend of hers who was to call me about a professional appointment, did not call. I told her that I was no longer upset at the situation because I now understand that it was one of three people who were trying to teach me a lesson in that week.

The first person was Cindy, who cancelled our dinner engagement two minutes before 6:00 because her roommate John was making her dinner at her place. The second was Carolyn replying to my email and saying that she would call me Saturday morning but did not. The third person was Bobbi, who was to call me at 6:00 p.m. to discuss our presentation that was due Monday. When Bobbi did not call at 6:00, I called her at 7:00, but she was not home. In all three situations I made arrangements, and these people did not live up to their ends of the bargain, leaving me at home alone waiting for them to keep their word and call. The lesson was that I must keep my word or promise to myself. If I don't respect my own words enough to keep them, then why should anyone else?

Patricia told me that a psychic had told her that even though she did not have a good relationship with her mother, she would when her mother died. I then told her that I had a better relationship with Mom today than when she was alive, because I talked to her all the time. She then asked me if I was still angry with Mom, and I said no and recanted the story of a Dru yoga assignment I once did. The lesson here was that Mom was telling me that I was on the right track in getting the colonics to clean up the toxicity within me. It was now time to release all that I was hording within my body and make room for the new.

Another great lesson occurred during the first two weeks of the life skills coaching program. I had the most difficult time with the instructor. Her motto was, "I will tell you what to do, and you will do it without questioning it." That did not work for me because I believe that those who don't ask for qualification of what they don't understand or agree with end up being worse off.

Each time she told me to act without questioning my mind, I went back to the Jim Jones mass suicide in Jonestown, Ghana. These suicides happened when the cult leader told his followers that they must drink the Kool-Aid and die, because God said so.

Soon after that, I realized that I have a lot in common with Natalie, including escaping into books as a child and being defensive when others criticize us. I still do today in the sense that when others criticize something that I am passionate about, I get extremely defensive and try to tune them out because I was not ready or willing to look into it, even though I needed to. She showed me that I sometimes put my head under the sand, pretending that the problem does not exist, while getting upset because others are right. I also escape life through going back to school instead of working when I am confused as to what direction to take. This is how I avoid living my life. When life gets to be too much, I go back to school to escape, which I disguise as finding myself and gaining knowledge.

This experience taught me that I am a very strong and powerful person, in the sense that I really do know what I like and don't like, what I want and don't want. To others it could be interpreted as arrogance and resistance to change, but nothing could be further from the truth. It's that I have strong convictions about what feels right to me and who I am as a person.

This strength is not always a welcome sight because it's scary for some people, so my lesson at the Private College was to learn how to contain it when necessary and when to pull it out. Natalie is afraid of strong-willed people, but she showed me what it looks like and what to do when others are afraid of power. It's about manipulation, of which she is a master.

I had a very difficult time at the Private College because they were asking me to compromise myself, and I was determined not to do so. The bullies' mission was to provoke others, causing an eruption in order to have something to fix. They wanted me to trust them, and I couldn't because I only trust those who are not trying to control me. I will trust you as long as you accept me exactly as I am.

I am fighting to keep me alive, whereas they are trying to break me down. All I wanted was to find the light that is the future, and all they wanted was to put me into the dark that is the past. I told them that in order for me to trust them, they would have to accept all that I am without judgment or reservation; they'd have to love me without wanting to change who I am. After making that statement, I realized that I was asking them to do the same that I have been resisting. We all want the other person to give in and accept our opinion wholeheartedly.

Why do I need to be the one who gives in? That's a question I ask myself when there is a difference of opinion or a conflict between another and myself. I realized it's because the greatest learning is in making someone else right, thus making them feel good about themselves, and because I am a leader and a teacher.

During my stay at the school I learned that in order for me to speak my truth and have others listen, I must set the stage for gaining the trust of the participants. Through my difficulties at the school, I realized that my lesson is in learning how to take care of someone else's feelings to make them feel safe opening up to me, so that I can get my point across in order to teach what they need to learn. By doing so I won't lose anything, but I will gain a lot in return for my patience and understanding of others. Some people are uncomfortable in dealing with calm and happiness, so they create chaos to feel better, wanted, and useful. The Private College provides me with the stimulus for these lessons.

At times I found myself in situations where I have asked for something that has been answered, and I have been pushing it away because of its package. It's not what I expected, so I don't recognize it and as a result push it away. For example, when I asked the universe to please give me the opportunity to go back to school and write full-time and my wish was granted, I had mixed feelings about it because it left me with no income.

I resist marketing myself because I used to believe that sales and marketing of the self is beneath me. It goes back to my early childhood of being treated as a princess who expected everything to be given to me without asking. I should just open my doors, and clients will come rushing through.

I found my self-confidence when I realized that I have the brains, the heart, and the courage for success—what was missing was direction in what to do next. I was extremely confused about what direction to take because of the many choices available to me. I always gave myself choices when I wanted to sit on the fence and not make a decision because of my irrational fears of success. This fear leads to binge eating, which shows up as an overweight body. I was resisting success because the *princess* in me was waiting for someone to come and take care of me. I am no longer waiting for anyone to prop me up, because I can do it all for myself. This princess is a huge success, now and forever.

The dysfunction of the class reminded me of my life during my teen years, when I felt abandoned, alone, and isolated. I was resisting letting down my guard and revealing the real me because I didn't feel accepted by the first few times when I was being myself. When I did say what was on my mind or disclose something about my past that was the absolute truth, they would say that there was more to it because it was not painful enough for them—meaning that because I was not crying during disclosure, I was holding back. I felt that the only way I could be accepted by Natalie and the group was to blindly accept what they were saying and asking me to do. They felt closer to me when I cried. I told them that I was not being me when I blindly did what I was being asked to do, but it fell on deaf ears.

I would love for them to listen to me for a minute, just to listen and acknowledge that they heard what I have said. They don't have to agree with me; they just have to listen. I have something to say, but no one wants to listen. What I would like to say, if I had an audience, is, "Please love me. Please accept me as I am, because I am doing the best I can. Please listen to me." I want to talk, and others just want me to shut up and agree with them. I feel that they cannot see me, and that's why they are not listening to me.

I get angry when others don't validate me and how far I have come. The fact that I have been working on myself and my feelings for 11 years prior to attending the Private College did not matter to them. It did not matter that I had healed old wounds by acknowledging them, forgiving all involved, and releasing them.

"If it's to be, then it's up to me" is one of my favourite quotes. I must validate myself and stop looking for validation from outside sources. I feel validated when others agree with me. Do I want validation or someone to agree with me? I must look for validation in what I do now. My frustration over the lack of validation is wrong. People can't validate me because they can't see or accept where I am now, because of where they are themselves.

Even though the Private College was not what I was expecting, I gained a lot of insight about how I interact with the world around me—and within myself as well. I learned that my blind spot is trying to avoid being put on display, and that I use speech as a weapon. I am using my weight as a cover to not live on purpose.

When you are straightforward and honest with me, I am open to your suggestions and ideas. However, if you are not, then I perceive you as judging me, which causes me to defend myself. Honesty is the thing I value most in others.

The biggest awareness occurred after what's called the power weekend. That's when the entire class spent the weekend at school without sleep, coaching and giving feedback to each other. I was not looking forward to it because of how the class had treated each other in the past. I did decide to keep an open mind by not thinking about it. To my surprise I came through it without a scratch—in fact, everyone was very nice to each other.

The Monday after the weekend, I was telling Steve, a former graduate, how the weekend went. I suddenly realized that I went into power weekend without expectations, and as a result I did not get hurt. Later that morning I realized that the reason I had such a difficult time with counselling and coaching class was because I came into this school extremely excited due to my preconceived ideas of how the programs would be. When it turned out to be the exact opposite of what I thought, I got extremely upset and confused about why I was there. I learned that it's not about changing someone; it's about understanding, because there are always two sides to each story. Listen with an open mind, without judgment or attachment to the situation.

I know I painted an unflattering picture of the Private College, and I would like to close by saying that the school's intentions were honourable. What I did not agree with was its method of teaching. I believe that you can teach without hurting your students. In talking to graduates of the program, some accepted it for what it was, and others like me were swimming against the current.

WEIGHT AND SPIRITUALITY

What Is Spirituality?

Depending on the religious belief of the person you are speaking to, the answer to the above question varies. Spirituality is often thought of as very deep feelings of belief that provide an individual or group with a strong sense of peace, life purpose, and shared connections about life. This spirituality can be expressed through prayer, meditation, and a personal relationship with a higher power, or God if you wish.

For me spirituality is the fuel that drives me and feeds my soul. I believe there is a creator of a greater power than myself, and I can turn to it for guidance in my time of need for directions and support.

Whether you want to admit it, we all believe in something. Christians believe in the teachings of the Lord God and Jesus Christ. Muslims believe in the teachings of Allah. Jews believe in the teachings of the Bible's Old Testament. Buddhists believe in the teachings and the reincarnation of the Buddha. And we must not forget about atheists, who do not put any faith into things they can't see. But I do believe they have faith in themselves and in science, which means they do believe in *something*.

When it comes to religion, I don't have a lot to say because I believe in spirituality instead of religion. In my frame of thinking, religion is the institution of belief, whereas spirituality is the act of faith in something beyond me. It's not something I have to think about; I was raised a Christian, and I agree with most of the teachings because it feels right on a personal level. I don't question the fact that there is a God I can't see; I simply know he exists.

I was raised a Christian and still believe in most of Christianity's teachings. However, as an adult I do have free will, and as such I explored both Judaism and Buddhism. In the end I integrated parts of all three faiths to form my personal definition of spirituality. Like me, you can choose who or what to believe in. There is no right or wrong answer. It's about what is right for you in this moment.

I know what you are thinking: "Althea, it all sounds great, but what does it have to do with weight management?" Everything! It's looking to someone or something you believe in during your time of need for guidance and support. It's your own personal mentor and cheerleader. Your belief system is what keeps you focused and on track for successful weight management, as well as other life decisions and directions.

Internal Guidance System

In the chapter on career, I touched on following the signs of the universe. This chapter expands on this thought process. Within these pages are numerous ways we can tap into the universal resources available to all of us who choose to believe. I call this the internal-guidance system.

Life provides us with the answers we seek; all we have to do is slow down and pay attention to what's happening in and around us. Then we will receive the answers to our questions plus directions for living a strong, lean, healthy, and balanced life. We spend a lot of time and money looking outside ourselves to psychics, astrologists, mediums, drugs, alcohol, and unhealthy foods instead of listening to out instincts, interpreting our dreams, looking at the way people are entering and exiting our lives, and understanding the obstacles that are sent to lead us along our paths.

Obstacles encourage movement and get us unstuck so that we can move forward in life. This then forces us to make the necessary changes. We need obstacles in our lives—without them, where would we be? Would we leave our safety nets? Would we be as quick to write the next line or to move on from the old?

The feeling of being stifled and unfilled is the universe's way of telling us to focus on the next step in doing what we know we must do. These challenges are training grounds for figuring out our life lessons and following the signs of the universe to complete the puzzle that is our lives. Whether you call them obstacles, challenges, or signs, this chapter is all about such guidance.

One realization happened on November 14, 2003, but the signs were set in motion the previous day, when I arrived home and found a cheque in my mailbox for $50. You see, I used 80 percent of my last paycheque to purchase clothes because I was leaving my job and wanted to use the discount before I left. I left myself with enough money for bus fare for two weeks plus groceries. I started to run out of money because instead of taking my lunch to work as planned, I was eating out to the tune of $20 per day. I was down to my last $20, which would be enough if I stopped eating out for a week. I was very surprised and excited to receive the cheque. That evening I decided to stop by the banking machine and see if I could deposit the funds. To my surprise I could, so I did.

After I left the banking area, I realized the craving that I had for bread over the past hour had gone away. I told myself that I didn't need or want bread at this time. While walking in the mall to get home, I went past SAJE, the store that carried essential oils and other aromatherapy products. I stopped to read the sign that listed all the ailments that aromatherapy could help. I asked the sales person what she recommended for PMS, and she presented me with two essential oils and asked me to smell them and tell her what I thought. Both oils reminded me of prementa, the berry that is used to make all spice in Jamaica. My family farmed the berries, and I helped harvest and prepare them for market. She then told me of the menopause remedy. When I put it to my nose to smell it, the essence went straight to my third eye.

I then recalled all the situations that brought me to this point. I got money that I forgot was coming. I deposited the cheque at the bank machine without difficulty. I went into this store that I passed twice per day five times per week for 10 months without interest. Alysha, the salesperson, mentioned menopause out of the blue. I bought the menopause remedy.

On my way home I came to the realization that the mood swings and cravings of sweets and breads, even though they occur one week prior to my cycle, were not due to PMS but rather menopause, because I have only been experiencing these symptom over the past two years, during the onset of menopause. Prior to this I did not have PMS symptoms. The message? I must find a way to deal with my menopause symptoms. Look within, because these feelings and mood swings are the symptoms of a deeper issue that is desperately trying to get out.

On January 29, 2004, while watching Oprah's 50th birthday special, I got very emotional because of all the love that she received from everyone. Then I asked myself, "How may I give of myself freely?" That night while saying my prayers, I asked the same question. A few seconds later I thought of a situation that occurred that day, and it brought a smile to my face.

Jessica asked me if I knew how to get to the bank. I told her to turn right out of the parking lot and then make a left at the light and drive; the bank would be on the left. We both cracked up laughing at the very bad directions I had given her. On the 30th I checked my email, and there was email from a man by the name of Brian who wanted more information about my services. This was my very first inquiry, and I was very excited and scared at the same time. I am giving of myself freely when I am having fun and being totally silly, because this puts a smile on others' faces. The message? I am taking myself too seriously. I must calm down and have more fun. This will result in me attracting more clients. I am giving of myself freely without noticing it, such as when I am fooling around with someone, smiling at a stranger, and coaching and counselling others.

Over the past 10 years I have been asking what my purpose in life is. Why am I so unhappy? Why am I stuck in the same routine day in and day out, like a hamster on its wheel not getting anywhere? I have come to believe that I am feeling this way because of my preoccupation in knowing the future instead of focusing on the present moment. I cannot see what's going on because I am focusing on me, me, me, instead of the universe and its plan for me. The message? "For me to walk by faith not but sight" (2 Cor. 5:7). Stop looking for solutions, and they will find you in the end. Trust in the universe.

The image that I have in my head of my life thus far is the picture of a country road. To me a country road has beautiful trees and flowers and animals on both sides. While driving the paved road, it then branches off into a dirt road without warning. The beautiful road becomes very bumpy. You then ask yourself, "Where am I, and how did I get here?" While driving along I keep looking around, trying to find someone who can help me to get back on the comfortable, paved road. I drive for miles and miles, and eventually I find someone to help at the right time. I wasted a lot of time waiting instead of enjoying the beautiful scenery. If I worry, help will show up; if I don't worry and enjoy the moment, help will still come. So why not just be in this moment and have a little fun along the way?

It was December 14, 2003—my 40th birthday, the day I had been excited about reaching for as far back as I could remember. I did not know why until that day. For my entire life I have been searching for the land of milk and honey. That day I realized that I had been living there this entire time. I did not recognize it because I was of the opinion that it was a place where I was a successful weight management specialist. I'd spend my working days studying, writing, and teaching weight management to women. I'd be working for myself and at my own pace.

What I have come to realize is that working as a retail store manager is exactly what I was to be doing at this point in my life. I now know that I am a very important person in this universe. Even though I can't yet see the impact that I have on the people that I come in contact with at work each day, I am here to serve them. It may very well be that the image of self and my life's purpose, outlined above, are correct; it's just not the right time, and I must learn other lessons before moving on. As mentioned above, this lesson is all about being patient and having faith, and all will be revealed in the tomorrows. Once I relaxed, my purpose as I imagined it came into being one year later. All I needed was to be patient and trust in the universe.

All the life challenges I have been experiencing over the past four decades, especially with my weight, happened as a result of my resistance to my truth. I learned the only way to rectify the painful situations is to accept my role as it is today in the universe. In each moment I am exactly where I'm supposed to be to learn and then receive one more piece of the puzzle to my success. I now know that the expectations of my career and personal life are due to being impatient and having a limited knowledge of myself and the purpose of my place in the universe. I accept my life now as it is, laid out by my destiny. I accept without attachment to the outcome that this is where I must be today. Where I go in the future is not my concern at this point; I am to concentrate on the here and now, which is where the happiness, joy, and fulfilment is because tomorrow is always a day away. If I am waiting for the future to arrive so that I can be happy, then it is quite possible that I won't recognize it when it shows up, because I'm too busy complaining and finding faults with today.

My struggles and challenges are all part of the preparation for the work I'm here to accomplish. This was evident on Thursday, February 12, 2004, when I reluctantly went out to pick up food for dinner. I noticed how beautiful the snow-covered mountains were. I then started to think of my belief that to me, mountains represent strength, and water represents movement.

I then asked myself, "If I had a choice of living by the mountains or by water, which would I choose?" My immediate answer was water, because I need movement to move forward in life and my work. I also thought that a man represents strength to me, so living by the water with my husband is the ideal world for me.

When I got to the restaurant, I was told that there was a 12-minute wait for takeout, so I decided to browse in the nearby drug store. I went to the computer department to ask questions about software that I was interested in getting.

On my way out of the store, a senior woman got to the exit at the same time, so I motioned for her to go first. She then looked at me and said, "When you are looking for something, you just can't find it." I left the store smiling. I then realized that I was not getting the answers to the questions that I had been asking the universe because I was trying too hard, which forced me to ask the wrong questions at the wrong time.

This interaction caused me see that the more I obsess over my lack of relationship, weight, and career, the more pain and confusion I experience. I simply need to be patient, watch, and listen for the signs. I then made the connection as to why I am still single, which is because I was not sure what I wanted in life from a man. I then realized that I am looking for a man of great strength and integrity. Knowing what I want and being patient is all I need to do for now.

We all have an internal guidance system that is in constant contact with us. Are you listening to yours? What is it telling you? Out of the blue, mine told me to move to Vancouver. I listened and moved to a place I'd never been, and I believe it was the best decision I've ever made. She told me to go back to school. I listened, and the money I needed to complete the program showed up.

Look Within

Signs can also come from your action or reaction to situations occurring in your life on a daily basis. When this happens, you may ask yourself, "Why me? Why not you?" The universe is trying to get you to look at changing a certain area of your life, such as looking at the reason behind getting angry over something that's small and unimportant. Here is an example of one such event. Kalmon Fisher, who is the president of my company, visited us on Thanksgiving Day 2003. I was very upset when I heard that he was going to visit that day. I was so angry that I could not move my neck the day before the visit; it was locked in place. I felt insulted that he would visit on a holiday, which showed that he did not care about his employees. I then convinced myself to get over it, which I thought I did until he walked into the store. I was furious due to the fact that he came in and did not acknowledge the holiday, which then brought all the anger back.

One week later, I was still angry with the matter and told everyone I knew so. I was then approached about joining another retail company, and the offer was too good to pass up, so I did. Months later I realized that anger had nothing to do with Mr. Fisher—it was about me needing an excuse to make a change with my career. This anger was the justification I needed to leave the staff I loved and who loved me without feeling guilty. I realized that being angry when someone is not in agreement with my ideas of how we should treat each other is a sign that I am looking for an excuse for changing my life's direction.

When I am not looking for a way out, I accept the opinions and viewpoints of others without judgment. I was angry because I felt out of control over the changes I knew I had to make with my career. I wanted to follow my path in life, but I was afraid of letting others down—that's what that anger was really about. I view Mr. Fisher and other individuals as teachers who are telling me something is wrong, so I should take a closer look at what I am reacting to, thinking, doing, and more important feeling in that moment.

Anger also prevented me from seeing the truth because I was too busy blaming someone else for my fear of moving forward. That fear was being fed by my mistrust of the forces of the universe. I tell myself that the information my internal guidance system is getting is a result of my mind playing tricks on me; if I knew which route or direction to take, then I would not have to stay here and listen to all this crap.

I was angry at myself for not being able to follow through on the decision I made about my life's direction, as well as not being committed to following through without guilt or attachment when I eventually make a decision. That's why indecisive people drive me crazy: they show me how I'm acting in that moment and situation. This indecisiveness causes me to doubt myself, my ability, and my belief system. This is evident when I start talking about my experiences with metaphysics and spirituality, and others tell me that I am stupid or that I don't know what I am talking about.

The lack of decisiveness or conviction to my point showed that I was not convinced what my position was, or whether it was correct or my absolute truth. If I don't believe in myself, then how can I expect others to believe in me? Trusting unconditionally is the key. If I trust myself, then others will trust and believe in me wholeheartedly without judgment, attachment, or prejudice.

Spirituality is all about having faith in yourself and your ability; however, when that faith is swaying, that's when you call on your higher power for help and support. Ask for the help you need to embrace who you are, what you are, and the decisions you have made. Asking for help is a sign of strength and confidence, *not* weakness.

Another way you receive diving guidance is through your chosen job or career. I have come to realize that all the retail companies I have worked for in the past provided me with all the knowledge I need in order to learn a particular life lesson. Below are my previous jobs, their challenges, and lessons learned.

The first job that I had was with Lizanne's Fabrics. I went there at age 18 for two weeks of work experience through school; it's now called a practicum these days. I enjoyed it, and at the end I asked Sue, the manager, if she was hiring. She said no but asked that I fill out an application form, and she would call me when something came up. A few months later she hired me. When I went away to college, I transferred from my hometown to a store in Toronto. I worked in several of their stores in the greater Toronto area for 4.5 years with very little advancement.

With each year I would become more bitter because I would see people with less experience than I had get promoted into the assistant manager's position, and I would have to train *them*. I did not understand this because my reviews were great, and there were no complaints from management, the staff, or customers. I asked for more training but did not receive it. I also asked the store manager if I could sit in on one of her interviews, but she said it would make the interviewee feel uncomfortable.

It was very clear that I would not be advancing in this company, so I left. Looking back, I am sure what turned them off was my attitude, in the sense that when someone new got promoted over me, I would become quiet and withdrawn, with a sour look on my face. Because of my immaturity level at that time, I did not know how to properly go after what I wanted, so as usual I turned to food for comfort. Food kept me calm enough to do a good job, but it silenced my internal guidance system from hearing the truth of what my next plan of action was to be.

The lesson? *Due to my immaturity level at that time, I was not able to ask for what wanted. Looking back, I am not sure if even I knew what I wanted. I was a good, reliable tasker and trainer, but I lacked the ability to communicate what I really wanted, which was the assistant manager's position. I realized that they did not really know what my goals were because I did not share them with my manager. I was expecting her to read my mind and anticipate my needs like Papa did when I was a child. At the time I believed that as long as I worked hard, they would notice and would offer the promotion.*

Over the next 17 years I worked for another eight companies with pretty much the same results. At Britannica I was totally bored because I had no interest in selling books or training others to sell. I love to buy and read books, not sell them. The result was my inability to effectively communicate my distaste with others regarding their ethics, comments, ideas, and thoughts. I then left and went to the UCS Group. There, my issue was my inability to communicate to Tony about his unrealistic expectations of the store and its hours of operation, so I left.

At Collacutt Luggage and Handbags, again I had no interest in sales generation, so I focused on tasks. The store did extremely well, and then Collacutt decided to sell the lease to Bentley. I did not agree with the company's philosophy of how a store was to be run, plus I did not like their inventory lines, so I left.

I then went back to the UCS Group, where I had very little control over the store because of the structure that was previously set up with the landlord. There was also no interest in position on my part, and I was unhappy with the location and did not know how to communicate this to anyone, including myself.

At Just Kids, my interest in the position was nonexistent, resulting in my unhappiness, which I blamed on the location, and again I did not know how to communicate what I was feeling to anyone. As strange as this might sound, I was thrilled when Just Kids went bankrupt. This meant that I had a legitimate excuse to leave—someone else was doing the dirty work for me.

The best company that I worked for to this point was the Gap; however, the result was the same because I still disliked sales generation and selling, resulting in me not leading by example and just delegating. After leaving, I went back to school. After I finished school, I found myself in another retail store. I guess old habits die hard. At La Senza there was less emphasis put on sales and more on customer service; however, the pace was extremely slow and the pay was low, so I left for yet another company when they came recruiting.

I went to Laura because I was being paid $5000 more for a lesser position. However, things ended up the same because I still disliked selling and hated the idea of a manager with a sales target. I felt it was an insult to ask a manager to compete with sales associates for sales. In my mind, managers manage and salespeople sell.

I understood why managers were given a person sales goal—the problem was that I wasn't interested in being a salesperson. Even though I was good at it, I found it boring and unchallenging. I worked for Laura in Toronto and was transferred to Vancouver at my request with the same end result, so I left again. At the Maternity Store the light bulb went on as to how much I dislike selling. For the very first time I actually acknowledged it to myself and shared it with others.

All these companies did not bring me fulfilment because I hated selling and sales generation through the "leading by example" method. Not leading by example resulted in poor communication skills with staff and bosses. I became a manager to get away from selling. However, retail has changed, and I realize that I must sell and switch roles with associates in order to gain their trust, respect, and desire to work hard for me.

Yes, I did end up changing my approach with the business to make my employer and employees happy; in the end everyone was happy—with the exception of me. All the stores I managed did extremely well with me as a store manager. I was able to increase profit and promote several people who wanted to advance their careers. In the eyes of all who knew me, professionally I was very successful. However, in my own eyes I was not personally successfully because I was not doing what I loved.

The lesson? It's very clear to me today that what I am is a communicator of my truth, and I pass on information to others. The delivery of my message is the lesson that I had to learn in retail in order to move on. This is what makes me happy, content, and joyous. Each time I sit down with a client to talk about her weight, issues I get more excited.

In my role as a store manager I was known as the "fix it" manager. I would go into a store and turn it around, making it profitable in a short period of time. It was not fulfiling for me because I was helping corporations instead of the individuals. I was hungry to connect with individuals on a deeper, meaningful, spiritual level. I became very skilled at identifying and fixing the store's issues; however, it was the people I wanted to help. I am a people person.

The Best Teacher

I was of the opinion that I must avoid certain situations and people because I must speak my truth, which appears to be venom sometimes. That's no longer the case. I now know that I must say what I'm feeling even though it's not always well-received. It's not that I cannot speak my truth; it's that I must be aware of who is ready to hear it. It's about knowing my audience when communicating the truth on weight management and its impact on overall health. The tools I choose to use are writing, coaching, and counselling. I don't have to say everything I am feeling because sometimes the message is just for me.

Once I learned this lesson, I had to leave Laura and go to the Maternity Store, because I needed Pam and Annette to push me out of retail and into purposeful living. My frustration with my job was because the universe was telling me that I was not living purposefully. A great way to get to know yourself and uncover your true mission is for you to ask yourself this very difficult question: "What lies have I been telling myself, and why?"

On Tuesday, April 20, 2004, while on my way home after another difficult day at work, I asked myself that question and was stunned when I uttered to myself that I was a very bad store manager. My lack of interest and commitment in what I was doing caused me great pain. I was bad in the sense that the more years that I spent on the job, the more disconnected I was from my real work as a weight management specialist. I was getting more and more disconnected from my real purpose. I came to the realization that I had mistaken hard work for dedication and commitment. This was why it was very difficult for me to get to work on time or even to get out of bed in the morning.

Sometimes you are not supposed to see what is going on; rather, it's a matter to be experienced. This statement really hit home for me that day. A few days later, I came to the realization that retail is not for me, that I am becoming more and more of an ineffective store manager because my heart is not into it. Retail is a bad fit, and that's why I get so frantic and overwhelmed when there are a lot of tasks to be done. I take over a store, make it great, and then lose interest. I focus on tasks because if all the tasks are done efficiently and on time, it will mask the fact that I am not interested in my position with this or any other retail company. I was totally confused because for the past five years I had been trying desperately to get into coaching and counselling others on weight management and emotional wellness.

Things are occurring almost daily to keep me in retail and away from a field that I believe will bring me piece of mind and the satisfaction of helping people in a more meaningful way. Knowing that, then, why can't I get out? Why do I feel trapped? Well, it's because the job must end for the work to begin. I can now move on with ease after I have learned the lessons. I needed to come to this realization before I could move on.

I know what I need to do and what direction I need to take; however, my intense fear of rejection prevents me from moving forward. My solution is to subconsciously manifest a conflict with my employer so that I can move forward. One such example is using Kalmon Fisher as an excuse to leave Laura.

It wasn't until months later when I realized that it was because I needed Annette's behaviours to expose my real feelings and intentions to move me forward and away from this profession. Annette was sent to help me, to push me forward. Each time she gets me upset, it's a sign for me to release stored anger and resentment that I have been burying with food as a result of being afraid of moving forward. She also showed me that I am paralyzed by fear, which is preventing me from sharing with others, moving forward, and making decisions. Fear is the lack of trust and faith in the process.

The Zen proverb states, "When the student is ready, the teacher will appear." That teacher was Annette, who taught me to look at my contribution to how people treat and react to me. She forced me into leaving retail by encouraging me to look at what I really and truly want in a career. I had to answer the question, "How may I serve?"

I must give thanks to the universe for sending me my foes, because without them where would I be? I could be stuck in the same boring existence, not knowing what to do next or where to go. Challenges are sent into my life to force me to make a change, because my present job is now completed and it's time to move on to my work.

When a new foe enters your life, ask yourself: "What are they here to teach me? What opportunities do they bring me? What opportunities are they offering me?" It may very well be that they are here to provide you with another piece of the puzzle, or instructions of how to find your way back home and how to live purposefully.

I have problems with staff because I am a vessel for them to work through their pain. That's the gift I provide them. In the end we all helped each other with our earthly lessons. I help myself by helping others.

I realized that the lesson at the Maternity Store was over when, on Monday, April 26, 2004, a friend called me at work and asked me how I was. I said fine, and she then asked me if I was sure. I started to laugh and said yes. She then told me that my laughing made her nervous. I told her that I was in such a good place in my life right now that all the other stuff did not matter.

On my way home from work, I recalled my conversation and realized for the first time that my job does not matter. What matters is that I am listening and following the signs the universe provides to move me on in carrying out my work. It was at that moment that I made the conscious connection that I am truly out of retail. I need people in my life with the same thought patterns for balance, connection, and mutual sharing. I want to relate on a mutual level of respect, on a soul level.

Over the years I have learned that what others think of you determines how they treat you. For example, at Laura the staff recognized my talents, ability, and work ethic, and they were impressed and welcomed it. At the Maternity Store, on the other hand, they saw these same things as competition and a threat due to the fact that they wanted what I had. I also learned that I am more receptive to the ideas and recommendations of people whom I do not recognize as a threat or competitor. Life's conflicts build character to provide the strength you need to move forward in doing your work. Without conflict, there is no growth; without growth, there is no strength.

As a result I am now taking responsibility for what is happening in my life today, such as Annette being defensive and looking to catch me doing something wrong. I learned that I lost control over the store because of my lack of interest in my position and the job. On a subconscious level, this is the only thing that I could think of for moving forward.

The more you think, the more conscious you become. The answer is within; all you have to do is be patient and it will surface. I also learned that when people are nauseating to you, it is because they are extremely passionate about what they do, and chances are you are you don't feel the same about what you yourself are doing. An example would be when lovers show each other deep affection, which shows you what you are missing. You are upset because you don't want to face your true feelings on the matter.

After leaving the Maternity Store to go back to school, my appetite decreased because going back to school was the right thing to do at the time; I let go of my anger and frustration at the job and myself. I was aware of what I was eating, when, and why. I'd found my food trigger and was more in the moment and with my emotions.

It all comes down to me moving in the right direction, resulting in me feeling connected and experiencing pure joy after accepting my true calling. The fight is over and the living has begun. I realized in the end how much career satisfaction affects my eating patterns and my overall health.

It's easier to see both the flaws and the good in others. The next time you react strongly to someone regardless of the situation, ask yourself, "Am I reacting to the way I feel about myself?" Then explore the topic further. In the end, it's not about eating to feel better, and it's not about buying and collecting objects; rather, it's all about absorbing and taking in the energy that the universe is offering. Just figure out what you want, and it will come later. Stop obsessing and worrying about how you will get there; just relax, and it will happen. "For we walk by faith, not by sight" (2 Cor. 5:7).

In the end I also realized that the source of my unhappiness is my constant quest to understand why Mom abandoned me. I now understand that when a child feels abandoned—whether it's real or perceived—it's because that invisible bond of love between a mother and her child was not formed completely, if at all. That leaves the child without the knowing of when they are loved. In my case, I was eating to fill up that space because that's what I was taught by my distant grandmother. Mother and child are bound by love through the heart during the early stages of life; this leaves the child feeling safe and content, with the freedom to move forward in the universe. It provides the child with proper boundaries that prevent addictions, whether it's eating, drinking, smoking, or criminal activity? The bond provides the child with validation of self-worth, leaving him feeling secure in the knowing that all things are possible. If you can dream it, think it, and then it's possible.

You may ask what the lack of connection with my mother has to do with my career, my weight, and other life challenges. The answer is everything. Disconnection is the absence of belonging. Feeling disconnected means that I did not feel like I belonged to anyone or anything. It is all about knowing who we are and having the confidence to go after what we want with vigour. The fact is that without this connection, it took me much longer to figure out who I was and where I was going.

In writing this chapter, what I have learned is that the universe will always provide me with the answers that I am seeking; all I have to do is stop obsessing, sit back, and relax, and all will become clear at the appropriate time. I need to be open to everything and be attached to nothing. That's what the universe is trying to tell me.

CONCLUSION

When I started writing *Beyond Weight Loss,* I set out to answer some questions. How many times have we told ourselves that we need to lose weight, only to regain most of it? What's stopping us from maintaining our successes? In the end, I realized it's because we put a lot of time and energy into losing weight without thinking of what will happen when the weight is finally off. We put a lot of blood, sweat, and tears into taking this weight off—now what?

This left me wondering, "Why is it we plan for weight loss and not how to manage our weight once we reach our goal?" After numerous years of struggling with managing my personal weight, I realized that there are as many ways of losing weight safely and effectively as there are overweight people in this world. On the other hand, there is only one way to maintain permanent weight loss, which is to live a strong, lean, healthy, and balanced life on your own terms.

You were successful in taking the weight off, which proves that you are committed to losing weight. Having a plan to keep it off is proof of your dedication to living a healthy life. It's important to have a plan—without one you will not know where you are going, and you will always be playing catch-up. Instead of focusing on what not to eat, focus on eating several healthy meals throughout the day. Then look at your life centres: Is this where you want to be? If not, focus on getting to where you want to be, and your weight will balance itself.

Oprah Winfrey is someone whom I look up to a great deal. One of her favourite Oprahisms is, "What I do know for sure is …" Millions of women throughout the world are overweight. What I've learned over the past decades as an individual with weight issues, and over the past 13 years working in the weight-loss field, is that weight is just the symptom, not the root cause of unhappiness. Obsessive food cravings are nothing more than a distraction from the truth of who we are, what we do, and what action we are to take in moving forward.

When it comes to weight management for me, what I know for sure is that it's not so much about willpower, diets, or even nutrition. Successful weight management is about facing the truth of who you are, what you are, and what you do. Permanent weight management is about you being ready, willing, and able to accept of your truth. When things happen, it's very tempting to use food as a way of coping.

This point became very clear after finishing all seven chapters and the introduction to this book. All that is left is this conclusion chapter. Each morning I would wake up as usual and open the computer, and my mind would be plagued with everything but writing. I was having trouble focusing on summarizing. I was resisting writing this conclusion because I was sad that this book was completed and ready for printing. I did stick to my guns by constantly asking why I was thinking of food when I was not hungry. "How am I feeling? What am I experiencing in this moment? What emotion am I experiencing?"

This led me to the realization that I was feeling extremely

angry, and I was still not sure why. I kept asking myself, "Why am I angry? Which life centre is out of balance?" My personal growth and development centre was out of balance. I then narrowed it down to the fact that I was not ready to put my baby to bed. This wonderful book that I had spent many months writing was now completed, and I was not ready to send it off to the printer.

Even though I did not know I was resisting at first, I stuck with my goal of writing each and every day no matter what. Even if it was just a couple of sentences, I wrote something. This was what I was committed to do, so I stuck with it because in the end I knew I would have a breakthrough.

What I do know for sure is that no matter what challenges come your way, you must stick with your goal of reaching and maintaining your strong, lean, and healthy body. At first it will take a lot of effort to stay on track; however, the more you stay on course and acknowledge your feelings in the moment, the easier it will get.

For many years I used food to escape my true feelings, to bury the things my mind did not want to deal with in that moment. It was how I chose to cope with life. I do get that in that moment it's not where we want to be, and yet we continue to suppress our thoughts, feelings, and beliefs with food instead of owning our feelings.

When we focus on weight loss, then we are addressing the symptom and not the cause. In talking about the road I've travelled and what I've learned, I turn to food in an attempt to bury my truth, which was reflected in the shape of my body.

Permanent weight management is all about constantly taking care of ourselves. Sometimes we need to pause for a few minutes and take a deep breath. We must know when to put ourselves first and the right time to help family and friends through their difficult times. Whether you are a few pounds overweight or clinically obese, we all got to this point the same way. We are taking on too much and must let go of all the excess baggage that's standing in our way of true and everlasting happiness. Figure out which life centres are out of balance, and once you correct the balance, you will find peace in your life. When we make a shift in perspective to focus on the cause of our weight gain and not its symptom, then we are facing our personal truths.